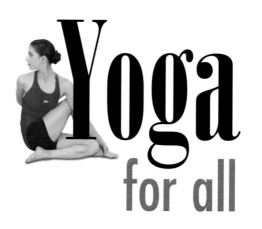

Yoga
for all

ISBN: 81-7436-215-0

© Bharat Thakur

Photographs: Deepak Budhraja, Abhishek Sharma

Published by
Roli & Janssen BV 2002
Published in India by
Roli Books in arrangement with
Roli & Janssen
M-75 Greater Kailash, II (Market)
New Delhi 110 048, India
Phone: 6442271, 6462782, Fax: 6467185
Email: roli@vsnl.com, Website: rolibooks.com
Conceived and designed at Roli CAD Centre

Printed and bound at Singapore

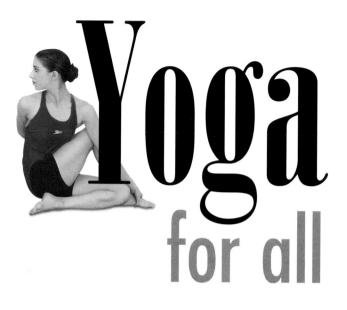

Yoga
for all

Text: Bharat Thakur

Photographs: Deepak Budhraja

Lustre Press
Roli Books

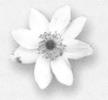

To my late mother and father
Abha and Dinesh Thakur

Contents

Introduction to Yoga   7

1   How Yoga Works   9

2   *Asanas* (Postures) – The First Step   15

3   *Surya Namaskar* (Sun Salutation)   19

4   Practising *Asanas*   25
   Legs • Hips • Sides • Upper Body • Back •
   Abdomen • Inverted Postures • Meditative Postures

5   *Pranayama* (Breath Regulation and Control)   101

6   *Kriyas* (Purification Techniques)   109

7   *Bandhas* (Restoring Hormonal Balance)   113

8   Meditation for Union of Body and Mind   117

9   Seven-day Schedule for General Fitness   123

10   Curing Ailments through Yoga   125

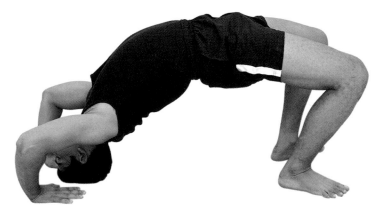

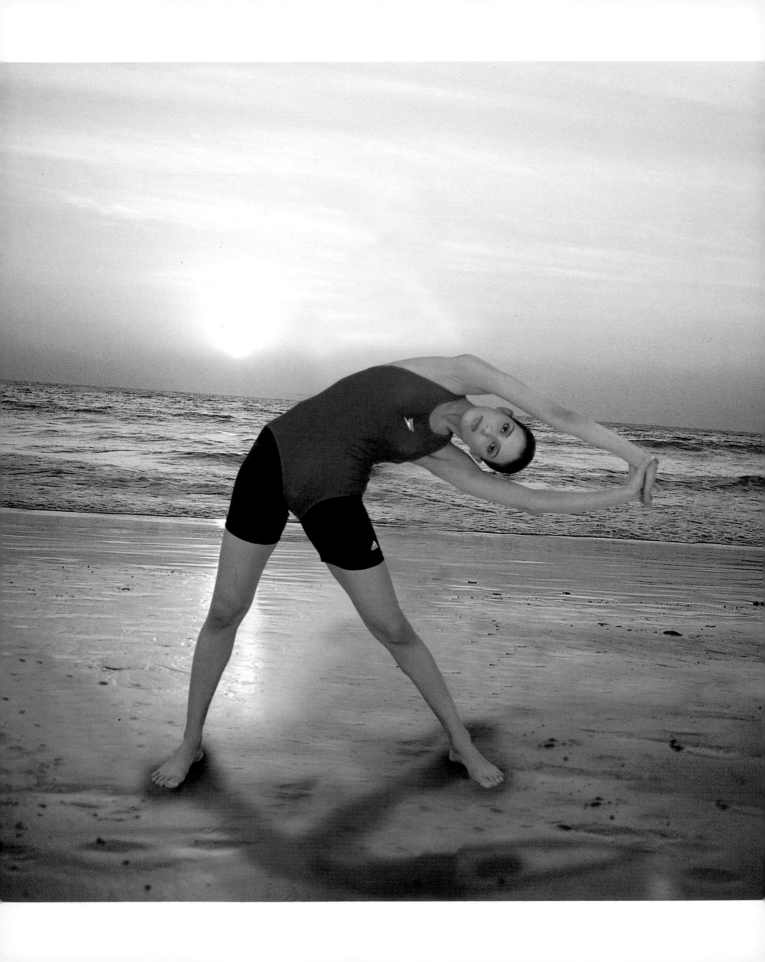

INTRODUCTION TO YOGA

Practised in India for thousands of years, yoga is more easily experienced than defined. It is neither a theory nor a philosophy, but a system that answers most of mankind's needs. If practised step by step, it has the potential to transform a human being at every level: physical, emotional, mental, and spiritual. It can do this because it recognises that these aspects are intrinsically connected and not separate from each other. Yoga is rooted in synthesis. Its approach is not to dissect, analyse, or deal with problems in isolation. It works at the very root of a problem and ensures that the body is able to correct and bring itself back into equilibrium. This is the beauty of yoga.

Aspects of Yoga

In ancient times, only yogis, sadhus or sanyasis, the first of whom was Shiva, practised yoga. Today, however, yoga has become one of the most popular forms of exercise or meditation and arguably, the best solution for stress management. It is the only form of exercise that not only involves the body and the mind, but also taps the higher centres of the human body called the conscious body, or the soul. The word yoga is derived from the Sanskrit word *yuj*, which means union – the union of the soul with the Almighty. It is also interpreted as the integration of each aspect of a human being – both internal and external. The sage Patanjali, credited as being the founder of yoga, describes it as yoga *chitti vriti nirodha*: a process by the help of which we can control the human mind and absorb right knowledge, erase the wrong, calm the mind, increase concentration, and sleep peacefully. Yoga can uplift one's concentration from one's body to the mind, and then to *samadhi* – the point at which man unifies with God. It is the only system that is free from any 'ism'. A person belonging to any belief system can move towards the ultimate goal of life – salvation – by practising yoga. This antidote to the stresses of modern living provides good health and a sense of well-being and fulfilment.

Today yoga is divided into several forms such as *asthanga* yoga, *hatha* yoga, *agni* yoga, *sahaj* yoga, *swar* yoga and others. But yoga as such is only one, which encompasses Shiva's research from concentration of the body to a *moksha shareer* (state of salvation). *Asthanga* yoga is divided into eight branches, hence its name. The eight stages are *yama, niyama, asanas, pranayama, pratyahar, dharana, dhyan,* and *samadhi.* When you step onto the first ladder, you automatically find yourself moving to the second, and so forth. The initial journey of yoga starts with *bahirang* (external) yoga, comprising *asanas* (postures), *pranayama* (breathing techniques), *kriyas* (cleansing techniques), *bandhas* (neuromuscular locks), and *mudras* (gestures). After that comes the second aspect of yoga called *antarang* (internal) yoga which consists of *pratyahar* (detachment), *dharana* (concentration), *dhyan* (meditation), and *samadhi* (state of bliss).

Yogis are researchers. The difference between a scientist and a yogi is that scientists research the external world and yogis research the internal world of man. Yoga not only exercises the physical body but also enhances the functional capacity of the whole brain. By practising yoga, yogis found that they were able to tap the higher levels of consciousness. However yoga is fundamentally an experiment conducted by oneself, on oneself, and the results are not always predictable. Every human being is different and each system has its unique qualities. During the course of your practice, you may find that your body or mind reacts to yoga in different ways. Since yoga works on the endocrine system, your body might go through several changes. This is natural as the body is simply being brought back to a state of equilibrium. But if your goal is not just to look good and be fit, you will need a master to guide you.

The Goal of Yoga

Yoga is the science of absolute freedom. It is the art of releasing, unwinding, and letting go till you reach a state of bliss. This peaceful state is achieved through constant practice of yoga and its principles of living. It works on the concept of beautiful living, starting from personal hygiene and physical fitness to emotional and spiritual freedom. It follows no beliefs, superstitions or laws. It is simply a set of guiding principles that leads you to a state of utter surrender to the divine. The final goal promised by yoga – that of *samadhi* – may seem abstract and strange at first. But yoga does not teach abstraction. It just takes you to the first step of the ladder, knowing that after the first step, you will automatically move to the second, and then to the third, and so forth. One starts by becoming aware of the body. Then the concentration shifts to breathing. After that, the functioning of the mind, with its weaknesses and its blocks, takes top priority. With *tapas* (effort), devotion and an experimental attitude, the practice of yoga helps one to move beyond the mind to a state of constant awareness and bliss.

1 How Yoga Works

Yoga is not only a form of physical exercise, which can benefit you by increasing your strength, endurance, flexibility, and sense of balance but can also help you in achieving spiritual enlightenment.

How Yoga Works

To understand how yoga works we need to understand how other forms of exercise work on the body. There are two kinds of exercises which are based on the intake of oxygen while being performed: aerobic and anaerobic exercises. The manner in which aerobic and anaerobic exercises affect the body is very different. During aerobic exercise, the intake of oxygen is very high. Activities like running, walking, dancing, and swimming are aerobic exercises that work mainly on the cardiovascular and muscular systems. Yoga is largely an anaerobic activity. It is generally performed with the minimum presence of oxygen. It is a complete system that improves not only the cardiovascular system with exercises such as *surya namaskar*, but also improves different aspects of the body such as hormonal balance, coordination and functioning of the organs, flexibility and strength of the muscles, to finally make a person active, agile, slim and glowing.

But how does yoga work? There are three kinds of exercises: isometric, isostatic, and isokinetic. Isometric exercises increase and decrease the muscle size due to which the muscle strength and shape improves. Isometric exercises, however, work on only one side of the muscles. For example, if you work on bicep curls, then the triceps are not dealt with. If you move the forearm upwards for the bicep curl, the downward movement of the forearm is a free fall. That is why the opposite group of muscles, which is the triceps, is not affected. This results in a waste of time and energy. Physiologists also figured out how to increase muscle strength in the shortest duration of time. They made computerised isokinetic machines for isokinetic exercise. If you do bicep curls with the help of isokinetic machines, the same amount of load is used to bring the forearm downwards as is used to pull the arm upwards. So the allotrophy (muscle size) of both muscles — front and back — increases very quickly. This form of exercise is today practised by the best health clubs all over the world. Indian yogis already knew of this concept. They had developed what is called an isostatic form of exercise — yoga — that was even more advanced than isokinetic machines. For example, to lift weights, you first have to know the optimum load you should use to begin the workout. Should it be five kilograms, ten or twenty? This involves spending much time and effort hiring a trainer or a specialist, thus making exercise an expensive proposition. Yoga, on the other hand, offers an inherent level of understanding as far as load is concerned. It maintains that the best load for a body is its own body weight. Since every person has a different weight, strength, and flexibility, each *asana* differs in terms of load for the individual. If you have a flexible body, forward bending and touching the toes is a basic load. On the other hand, if your body is stiff, this load can be intense and powerful because the stretching levels of the muscles are much higher.

Similarly, since holding a posture is the final step of each *asana*, you can vary the load by increasing and decreasing the duration of holding the posture. In terms of endurance, which is the basis of developing strength and flexibility of the body, exercises like *surya namaskar* (sun salutation), along with the number of repetitions and the speed of the movement, can also become part of load adjustment. If you want to develop cardio-respiratory endurance (ability of the heart and lungs to perform well for a longer duration of time under a given load), you can increase the speed of the *surya namaskar*, by which the efficiency of the heart and lungs can improve to a great extent.

The working of yoga, therefore, simply depends on what exactly you are looking for from it. If you look at it as a form of physical exercise, it can benefit you by increasing your strength, endurance, flexibility, and sense of balance. If you look at using yoga for achieving spiritual enlightenment, then the entire approach would change. All the 840,000 postures aim at mastering one posture out of the meditative postures, so that you can sit down to meditate for as long as possible without any stiffness or pain in the back or other part of the body. This is essential because the whole body needs to cooperate in order to allow a person to focus at one point.

Yoga and Body Systems

Endocrine System

Yoga affects the various systems of our body in different ways. The Endocrine System deals with the glands and its different secretions in the body for better metabolism and growth. Yoga aims to improve just this one and only one system which, in turn, will benefit the rest of the systems. How you look depends on the secretions of the different hormones in the body. If you are under stress, or aging prematurely, or diseased – this is probably due to the malfunctioning of the endocrine system. Whenever you practise a posture, be it an *asana*, *bandha*, *kriya,* or a *mudra*, you are pressing a particular gland in your body. As all the glands are porous and unidirectional in nature, whenever there is any pressure, they release certain hormones or juices. For example, if a balloon is filled with water, and many holes are made in it, the water comes out, a few drops at a time, from the side. If, however, the balloon is pressed, the water pours out with far greater pressure. In isometric and isokinetic

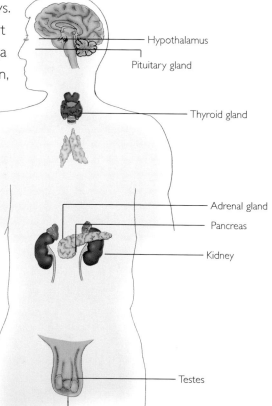

The major endocrine organs of the male body. The hypothalamus in the brain controls the activity of the pituitary gland.

Hypothalamus

Pituitary gland

Thyroid gland

Adrenal gland

Pancreas

Kidney

Testes

exercises, the hormones roll from the side, whereas in yogic exercises, they ooze out like a fountain. So while most followers of isometric or isokinetic forms of exercise look muscular with a good physique, they lack a glow on their skin due to one simple fact – isometric and isokinetic exercises believe in energy breaking, while yogic exercise believes in energy conservation. If you get tired while practicing *asanas*, yoga advises you to lie down in a resting posture or *savasana*. (Lie down on your back with feet apart, hands by your sides and eyes closed. Inhale and exhale deeply – see page 120). In fact, some yogic scriptures actually suggest that *savasana* is done after every two or three *asanas*. Some people find the working of yoga difficult to understand. They do not believe that yoga can make a person slim or flexible. What needs to be understood is that yoga does not depend on how many calories are burnt. It depends on how much the functioning of the endocrine system of the body can be enhanced. If the glandular secretions are increased, then the basic metabolic rate as well as the entire internal environment of the body automatically changes.

Circulatory System

Most diseases relating to the heart pertain to the Circulatory System. This is simply an indication that the circulation of the blood in the body is not right. One way to correct this is to perform aerobic workouts, which increase the heartbeat, which in turn, increases the force of blood circulation. Yoga uses a different approach. Instead of increasing the blood flow by force, it affects this circulatory system in a more uniform and relaxed way. To explain this, let us understand how reflex action works. If, by mistake, one finger of the hand touches a hot surface, the entire arm automatically jerks away from the surface, with the rest of the body. This reaction takes place in a cycle: first, a sensation is felt; this sensation then travels through the nervous system with the help of nerves present all over the body, and then comes the reaction. The brain informs the concerned group of muscles to rush and perform an activity as soon as possible. So the blood rushes there to supplement and give the required amount of energy to that part of the body to move away from the hot surface. Yoga works on the circulatory system in a similar manner. While performing any yogic technique, the brain recognises the contraction of the muscles, and immediately instructs the circulatory system to allow the blood to rush to that part of the body where the muscle is

Anterior view of the heart and the main arteries (red) and veins (blue) of the head, right upper limb, and the trunk.

being contracted, to release out the required amount of energy. This simply means that blood is shunted from the whole body to a particular body part. Consequently, when there is powerful circulation of the blood towards one part of the body, the flow of blood to that body part will automatically be rich, and, in turn, will clean out all the blockages present in any blood vessel in that area. Yoga offers an exercise for each muscle in the body, whereas aerobic exercises cater only to the longer muscles. By stretching and contracting different parts of the body, the whole circulation of the body becomes smooth and active.

Skull

Rib

Vertebral column

Pelvic (hip) girdle

Femur

Anterior view of the full skeleton.

Skeletal System

The Skeletal System includes joints, ligaments and attachments of muscles to the joints. The joints in the body have an important function that has to be understood in the working of yoga. There are stretch receptors present in the muscles and joints of our body. These are called propreo receptors, which analyse the degree of stretch to the muscles in connection with the joint. Stretch receptors consist of two organs: golgi tendon organs and muscle spindles which are connected to the ligaments and muscles of the body. Whenever you perform an *asana*, there is a tremendous stretch on one muscle group. These organs analyse the degree of stretch and inform the central nervous system. Accordingly, the brain starts registering the new stretches slowly, and allows the joints to improve their range of movement day by day. The stretch receptors also assist in reporting these at the muscular level of the brain, and the brain reacts by secreting hormones and juices which help with the growth and the metabolism of the body.

Brain

Cervical spinal nerve

Spinal cord

Lumbar spinal nerves

Nervous System

The Nervous System comes into play completely and fully while performing a yogic technique. Keeping a posture in mind, it commands the body to move effortlessly from one position to the next and finally to the main posture. The steps leading to the final posture are as important as the final posture itself. Eventually the mind is brought to a state of stillness and blankness. Yoga also teaches you to be aware of your breathing in every position, till you reach the final position. When the muscles of a particular body part contract, the neuroreceptors present in every body part, inform the brain about the entire activity. The brain, in

Sciatic nerve

The nervous system extends throughout the body The brain and spinal cord receive and send out messages along the nerves.

turn, starts working for the body part fully and actively, gradually moving away from absorption of knowledge and information, sleep, dreams, imagination, and ignorance to a focused state, and finally, all the neuro transmitters in the brain totally relax. A practitioner of yoga slowly learns the art of disconnecting from *the thought* to the *no-thought* stage, and in an advanced stage of *sadhana* or practice, remains in that relaxed blissful state even when *asanas* are not being practised.

Digestive and Excretory System

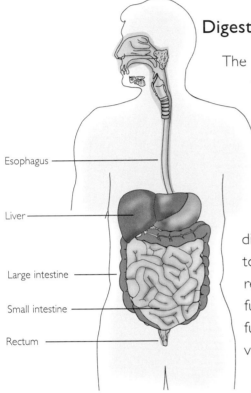

Esophagus

Liver

Large intestine

Small intestine

Rectum

Most digestive organs are located in the abdomen, as seen in this anterior abdominal view.

The Digestive and Excretory System are both positively affected by yoga. The digestive system includes the alimentary canal, from the oesophagus down to the stomach, the small intestine, large intestine, and the rectum. Yogis believe that to have a smoothly functioning digestive system, one needs to clean the internal organs too. Yoga offers several techniques of cleansing the whole alimentary canal, which results in healthy digestive and excretory systems. Certain *bandhas* and *asanas* activate the secretion of digestive juices, thus benefiting the entire digestive system. Yoga helps to tone the skin, thereby improving the capacity of each skin pore to release toxins in the form of sweat. This results in a smooth functioning of the excretory system. It also improves the kidney function which helps in renal filtration of the urine and the blood very actively.

Anti-aging and Yoga

Anti-aging and yoga are closely connected. Yogis look young even when they turn old because yoga involves less wear and tear of muscles. The muscle tone remains untouched, leading to a very healthy skin. Yoga increases the antigens present in the body, and consequently the ability of the body to fight against disease. As described above, if all other systems work smoothly, the immunity of the body is automatically high because there are less toxins in the body. This prevents the body from falling sick. In each animal cell, there is an organ called lysosome, whose function is to absorb the unwanted things in the body. The functioning of the lysosome is found to be more efficient with the practice of yoga. Aging is merely a state where the dying cells are greater in number than the new cells being formed. Yoga stops the cells from dying and helps to enhance the growth of new cells, thus keeping the body toned and youthful.

Yoga works not only at the muscular level but at all levels of the body, to ensure that every aspect of the body's functioning is smooth, balanced and in equilibrium.

2
Asanas (Postures)
The First Step

An *asana* or posture is a combination of movements that leads one into a final posture. Each movement works on your body by contracting specific muscles, and extending or stretching other muscles. The correct breathing is an important aspect in the practice of *asanas* and regulating the breath is important to nourish the body with plenty of oxygen.

What are *Asanas*

Asanas are the first step of the physical aspect of yoga. Patanjali describes them as *sthiraha sukham asana* which means any posture taken for stability and a feeling of well-being. *Asanas* should be performed effortlessly by focussing the mind beyond — to the breath, to the body parts in action, or to any external music. The goal of all *asanas* is to ensure that every part of the body is flexible and strong. And finally, to bring harmony between the body and mind so that the awareness can move from the physical body towards higher levels of consciousness.

Forms of *Asanas*

There are three forms of *asanas*.

Cultural *asanas* — to strengthen and tone the muscles.
Meditative *asanas* — to move from awareness of the physical body to awareness of the consciousness.
Relaxing *asanas* — to relax the body and rejuvenate it.

All three types of *asanas* need to be practised for the body to improve in a smooth and steady manner. The right combination of these three types of *asanas* ensures that the body remains healthy, light, and energised.

How *Asanas* Work

An *asana* is a combination of movements that leads one into a final posture. Each movement works on your body by contracting specific muscles, and extending or stretching other muscles. To support a posture the body functions through two muscle groups — antagonist and agonist. For example, when you bend your arms from the elbows, the biceps become agonist and the triceps become antagonist. *Asanas* should be performed for both groups of muscles, agonist and antagonist. If you do a forward bend posture, it should be followed by a backward bend. A posture should be held as long as possible, but if you lack the strength, you can perform each posture twice or thrice until you gain the strength to hold it for a longer duration of time. Breath is an important aspect in the practice of *asanas*. Normally, one breathes in a shallow manner, not inhaling large amounts of oxygen rich air and not fully exhaling the unwanted air from the lungs. Regulating the breath is important to nourish the body with plenty of oxygen. This also ensures that residual air inside the lungs is removed. Performing *asanas* well results from a combination of focussed movement and awareness of the breath at all times.

When one starts yoga by performing *asanas*, one moves from a diseased state of the mind called *vikshiptachitta* to a blissful state of the mind called *ananda maya chitta*. Initially when you practise *asanas*, you will have tremendous body vibrations. For example, if you raise your leg, your whole body starts to tremble because your muscles lack strength. Yoga refers to this initial stage as *aangamaya* (bodily vibrations) which would lead towards *asanajaya* (a relaxed state of the muscles even under tremendous contractions).

Practicing *Asanas*

The conditions under which one practises *asanas* are as important as the posture itself. The aim of *asanas* is to ultimately bring about stillness of the mind. And this can happen only under suitable conditions. Keep the following points in mind when you practice *asanas*.

▶ Choose a quiet space with plenty of sun and fresh air.

▶ Wear loose comfortable clothes, or skin tight clothes for ease of movement, preferably cotton.

▶ Yoga should be practised on an empty stomach. Avoid eating at least two hours before the practice.

▶ Yoga can be practised for twenty minutes, forty minutes or five hours a day depending on one's need.

▶ Try to maintain a posture as long as possible, from ten seconds up to a minute.

▶ Try to practise *asanas* on a yoga mat or any cushioned surface.

▶ Breathe normally, except where indicated. In general, inhale while bending backwards and exhale while bending forwards.

▶ Practise yoga six or seven days a week. A day's rest can be taken.

Consult your physician before starting yoga if you have any specific medical problems.

Schedule

Given at the end is a seven-day yoga schedule that can be practised throughout the year.

Surya Namaskar Cycle
Sun Salutation Cycle

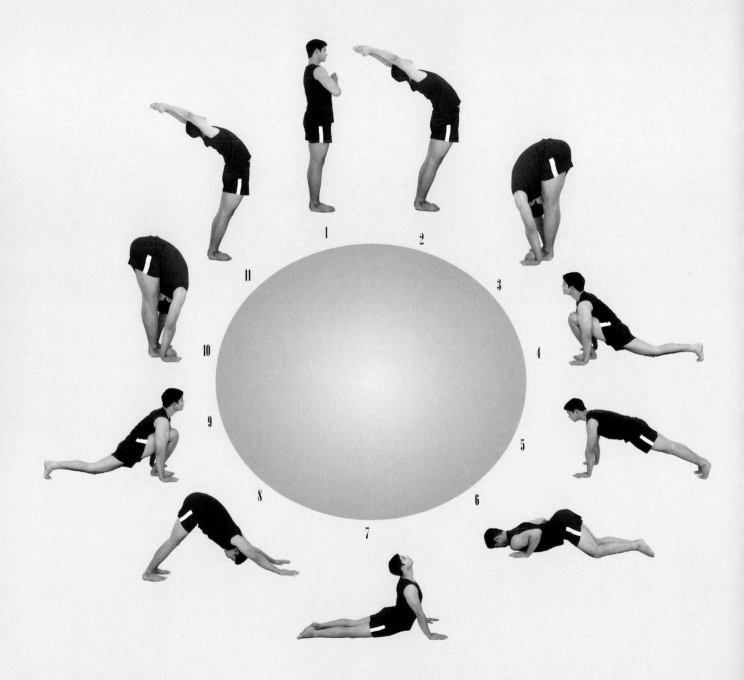

3

Surya Namaskar

Surya namaskar or sun salutation, is a combination of eight *asanas* usually done to warm up before practising and performing other *asanas*. This *asana* affects practically every muscle of the body, and practising this regularly ensures good health, flexibility and strength.

Surya Namaskar
Sun Salutation

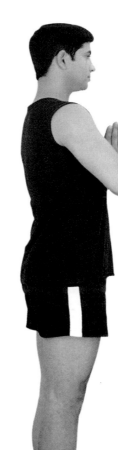

1 Stand straight with feet together and palms folded in front of your chest. Breathe regularly.

2 Inhale and stretch your hands over your head locking the shoulders and the ears together and bend backwards.

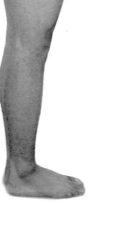

3 Exhale and bend your body forward till your fingers, palms or hands touch the floor by the side of your feet. Touch your knees with your forehead and relax.

4 Inhale, take your left leg back and place both your palms on the floor on either side of your right leg. Arch your back and avoid touching the floor with the left knee.

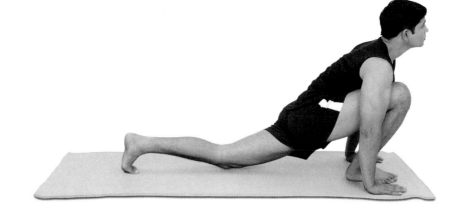

5 Exhale and take the right leg back and make a straight line from head to toe, the body weight balanced on the toes and palms.

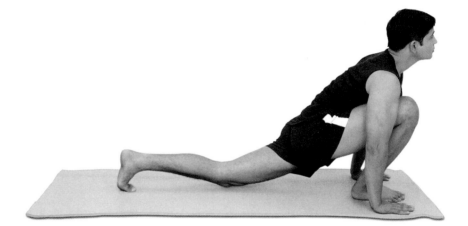

6 Hold your breath and place your knees on the floor, then bend your elbows and press your chest and forehead on the floor. In this position your toes, knees, chest and forehead touch the ground.

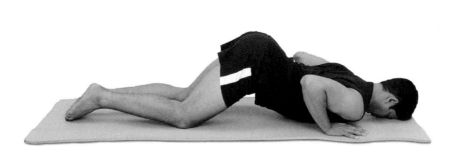

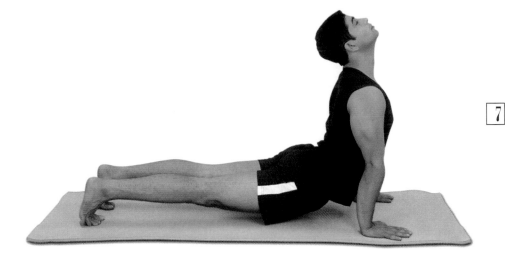

7 Inhale and stretch your trunk upwards. Straighten your elbows and arch the back to look up.

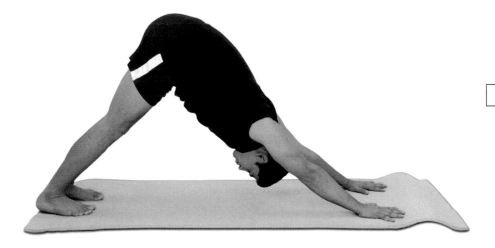

8 Exhale and raise your hips upwards as high as possible tucking the chin inwards towards the chest looking at the navel. Your heels remain pressed flat on the floor.

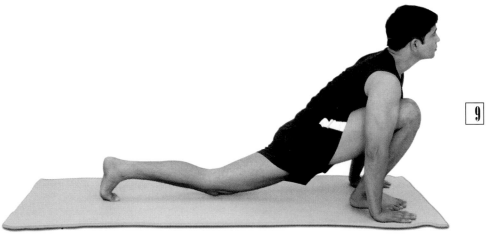

9 Inhale and bring your right leg forward arching the back.
Note: In subsequent rounds alternate between left and right leg in Step 4 and Step 9.

10 Stand upright, exhale and bend forwards to touch your toes as in position 3.

11 Inhale and stretch your hands over your head and bend backwards as in position 2.

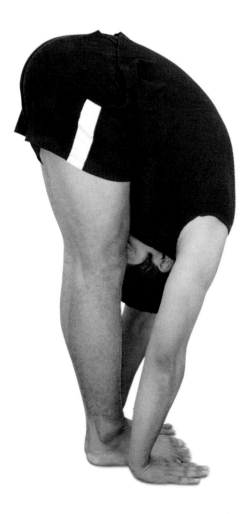

24

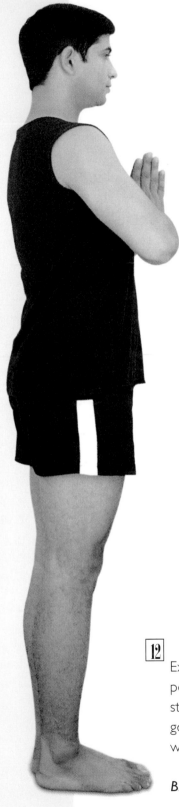

Benefits

- Improves the flexibility of the whole body
- Improves cardio-respiratory endurance if done at a quick pace
- Effective in weight loss
- Opens the *granthis* (the physical blockages of the body) and makes it look younger, vibrant and glowing
- Improves the autoimmune system
- Balances all the vital plexus of our body from the *mooladhar* (the root plexus) to the *brahamarandra* (the crown plexus)

Caution

- Those suffering from high blood pressure, stroke, weak heart, hernia and severe back problems should not practise this

12 Exhale and come back to position 1. Repeat this cycle starting with 10 rounds and going up to 51 or 101 rounds within 2 or 3 months.

Breathing: Normal

4

Practising *Asanas*

Legs • Hips • Sides • Upper Body • Back • Abdomen •
Inverted Postures • Meditative Postures

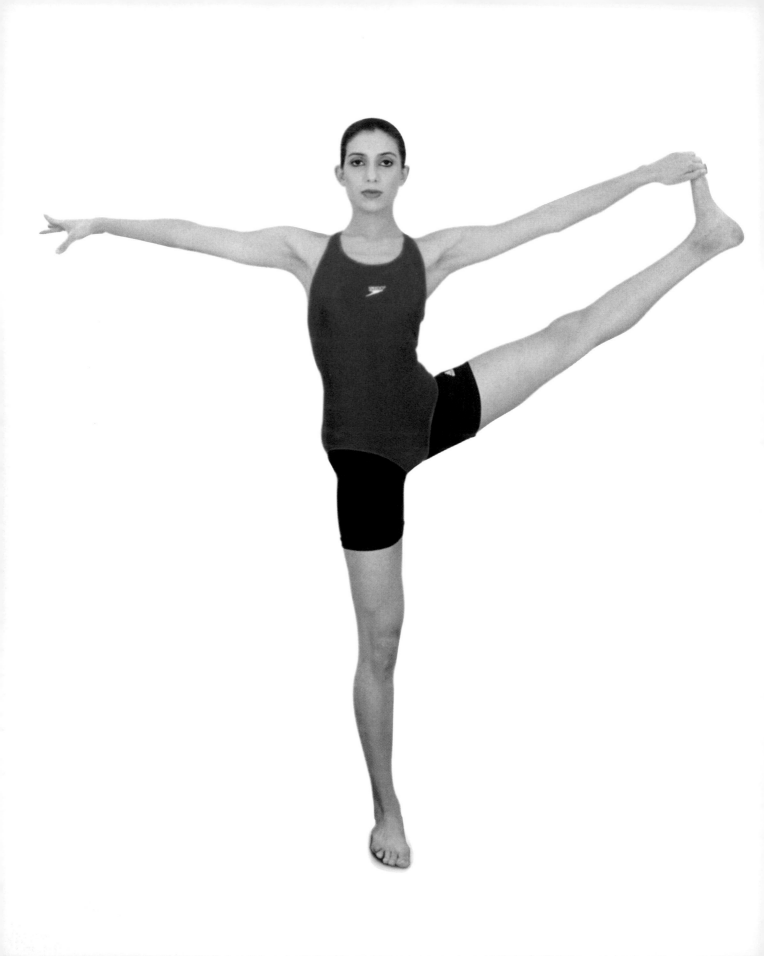

LEGS

These *asanas* work specifically on the hamstrings, quadriceps and calf muscles, and also strengthen the ankle and knee joints. Practised regularly, they will tone and shape your legs, improve your figure and make your body swift and agile.

Uthita Pada Uttanasana
Front Leg Raise

L E G S

Stand with your feet together balancing the body weight on both feet. Slowly raise one leg off the ground straight in front. Bring your arms forward parallel to the ground and hold the posture for 10–30 seconds.
Repeat with the other leg.

Breathing: **Normal**

Benefits

▶ Strengthens the muscles of the legs

▶ Improves the sense of balance

▶ Improves concentration and neuro-muscular coordination

Cautions

▶ Those with knee joint pain should avoid standing for a long time

▶ Those with varicose veins should not practise this

Uthita Kona Pasa Uttanasana
Side Leg Raise

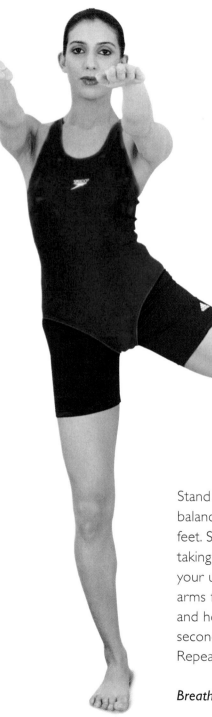

Benefits

▶ Strengthens the muscles of the legs

▶ Removes excess weight from the outer sides of the thighs

▶ Strengthens and tones the hip muscles and lower back

Cautions

▶ Those with knee joint pain should avoid standing for a long time

▶ Those with varicose veins should not practise this

L E G S

Stand with your feet together balancing the body weight on both feet. Slowly raise one leg sideways taking it as high as you can. Keep your upper body straight. Bring your arms forward, parallel to the ground and hold the posture for 10–30 seconds.
Repeat with the other leg

Breathing: Normal

Virabhadrasana
Hero's pose

**L
E
G
S**

Benefits

▶ Strengthens the legs and the knee and ankle joints

▶ Reduces fat from the hips

▶ Improves the functioning of the abdominal organs

▶ Relieves stiffness of the shoulders, back and neck

Cautions

▶ Those with heart problems should not practise this asana

▶ Those with high blood pressure should not practise this asana

1   Stand with your legs together, arms above your head and palms together. Turn to the left, bring your left foot forward, placing it 4-5 feet away from the right foot. Bend the left knee, until your left thigh is parallel to the ground. Bend backwards and look up. Hold for 10 – 30 seconds. Repeat with the other leg.

Supta Vajrasana
Reclining Hero

Benefits

▶ Strengthens and improves the flexibility of the ankles and knees

▶ Stretches the front of the thighs and makes the quadriceps flexible

▶ Improves the posture of the back and the curvature of the spine

Caution

▶ Those with back and neck problems or with stiff ankle and knee joints should not practise this

**L
E
G
S**

1

Sit in *vajrasana* as above (kneeling position with your buttocks on your heels), slowly bend backwards taking the support of first one elbow and then the other. Hold your ankles with your hands and arch your head back.

**L
E
G
S**

2 Slowly lower your back and head to the ground as you hold your ankles with your hands. Try to keep your knees on the ground.

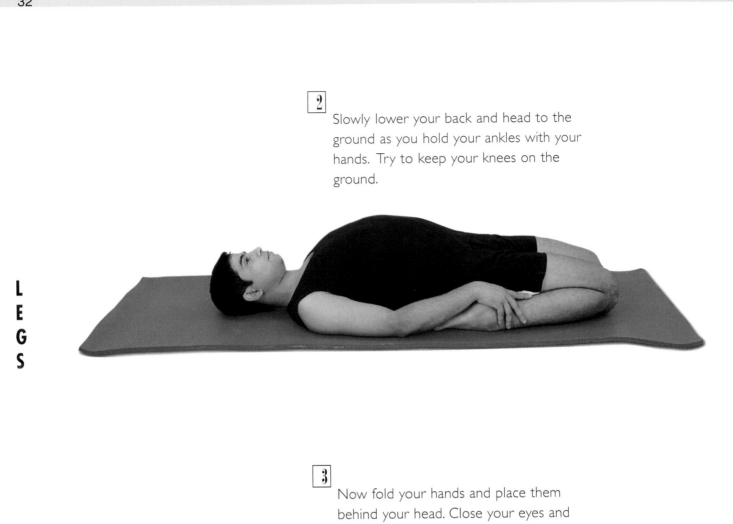

3 Now fold your hands and place them behind your head. Close your eyes and relax in this posture for 10–30 seconds.

Breathing: **Normal**

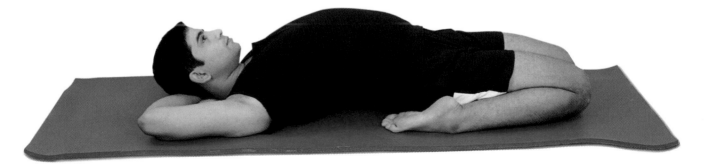

1 Stand with your feet far apart and your hands on your waist.

Natarajasana
The Statue

L
E
G
S

Benefits

▶ Strengthens the thigh and calf muscles

▶ Strengthens the ankle joints

▶ Removes excess weight from the sides of the thighs

▶ Improves the posture and sense of balance

Caution

▶ Those with stiff knees and ankles, or with a weak back should be careful while practising this

2

Bend your knees, keep your back straight and stretch your arms straight above your head. Join the palms together and hold the posture for 10–30 seconds.

Breathing: **Normal**

Padahasthasana
Fan Pose

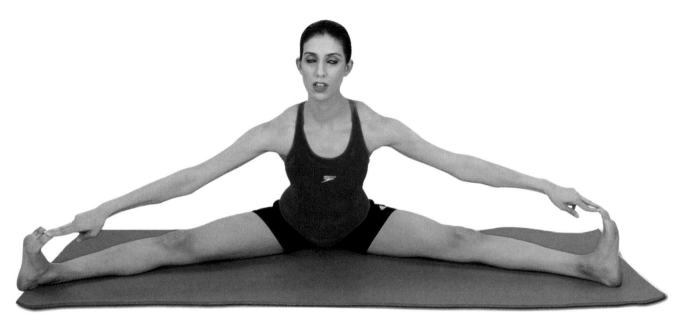

Sit on the floor with your legs split sideways.
Keep your back straight and hold your toes with
your hands. Hold the posture for 10–30 seconds.

Breathing: **Normal**

Benefits

▶ Brings flexibility to the groin
▶ Stretches the inner thighs and reduces
weight from the hips
▶ Improves the flexibility of the lower
back

Caution

▶ Those with a weak back or
suffering from hernia should not
practise this

Ek Padakonasana
Moon Pose

LEGS

Benefits

▶ Shapes the hips and thighs
▶. Stretches the hamstring
▶ Improves the sense of balance
▶ Strengthens the legs

Caution

▶ Those with varicose veins or suffering from vertigo should not practise this

Stand with your feet together with your arms outstretched sideways. Slowly raise one leg sideways and hold your toe with your fingers pulling your leg upwards as high as possible. Keep your spine straight and hold the posture for 10–30 seconds.
Repeat with the other leg and arm.

Breathing: **Normal**

Sahaj Vyagrasana
Half Crane Pose

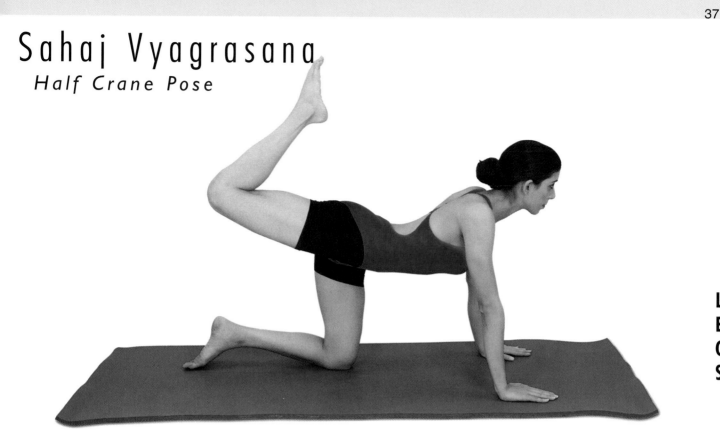

Kneel on a mat or cushion on the floor. Bend forwards
resting your body on the palms of your hands and look
straight ahead. Avoid bending your elbows. Raise one leg
and stretch it straight out parallel to the ground. Hold
the posture for 10–30 seconds.
Repeat with the other leg.

Breathing: **Normal**

Benefits

- ▶ Strengthens the back, thigh and
  buttock muscles
- ▶ Strengthens the arms
- ▶ Removes fat from the hips
- ▶ Alleviates cervical spondylitis

Caution

- ▶ Those with high blood
  pressure or severe back
  problems should not
  practise this

Vatayanasana
Arched Moon Pose

Benefits
▶ Strengthens the knee joints and the muscles of the legs
▶ Reduces fat from the hips
▶ Strengthens the back

Caution
▶ Those with knee problems or varicose veins should not practise this

1 Stand with the left leg behind the other, its heel off the ground and the left arm hanging down the side. Raise the right arm straight up. Inhale and slowly raise the left foot behind and hold the toes with the left arm making a triangle between your back, arm and leg.

2 Exhale and bend your torso forward, and lower the right arm in front of you till it is parallel to the ground. Balance the body on the right leg still holding the left foot with the left hand and hold the posture for 10–30 seconds. Repeat this exercise on the other side.

Breathing: **Normal**

HIPS

These *asanas* work specifically on the buttocks – the gluteus maximus and gluteus minimus muscles. Practised regularly, they will tone and firm up the buttocks, give additional mobility and flexibility to the hip joints and improve your gait.

Paschimottanasana
Forward Bend

**H
I
P
S**

Benefits

▶ Stretches the hamstring muscles

▶ Helps to remove excess fat on the thighs

▶ Increases the flexibility of the hip joints

Caution

▶ Those with lower back problems should not practise this

Sit on the floor with your legs stretched in front, feet together. Slowly exhale and bend forward from the hips trying to hold your heels (or toes) with your fingers. Touch your forehead to your knees, your elbows resting on the ground and hold the posture for 10–30 seconds.

Breathing: **Normal**

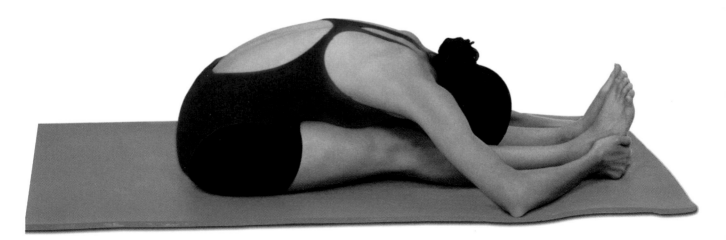

Hastha Padasana
Forward Stretch

Stand with your feet together and back straight. Exhale and bend forward from the waist, to touch your knees with your forehead, arms holding the back of your ankles. Hold the posture for 10–30 seconds.

Breathing: **Normal**

**H
I
P
S**

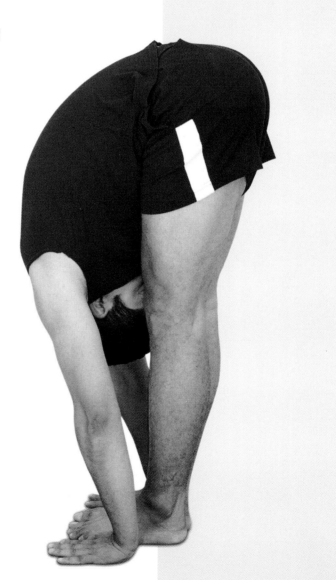

Benefits

▶ Massages and tones the abdomen
▶ Opens up the hips and stretches the hamstring muscles
▶ Increases blood flow to the head, improves metabolism, concentration and vitality

Caution

▶ Those with high blood pressure or severe back problems should not practise this

Swastik Padang Ustrasana

Knee Bend Leg Raise

**H
I
P
S**

Go down on your hands and knees looking straight ahead. Slowly raise one leg above the ground and fold the knee upwards. Hold the posture for 10–30 seconds.
Repeat with the other leg.

Breathing: **Normal**

Benefits

▶ Strengthens and tones the legs
▶ Strengthens the back muscles
▶ Strengthens the gluteus muscles (buttocks)

Caution

▶ Those suffering from excessive lower back pain should avoid raising the knees very high and bending the arms

Hastha Moordhasana
Wigwam Pose

Stand with your feet wide apart.
Bend forward from the waist till
your hands touch the ground.
Hold your body parallel to the
ground. Keep your back straight
and look ahead.
Hold the posture for 10–30
seconds.

Breathing: Normal

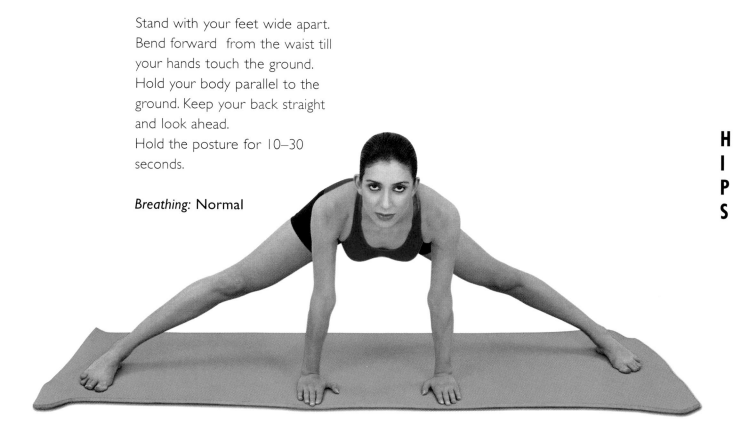

Benefits

▶ Helps to remove excess fat on the
calves, thighs and buttocks
▶ Improves flexibility of the back
▶ Strengthens the arm muscles
▶ Removes stiffness from the hip joints

Cautions

▶ Those with lower back problems
should not practise this
▶ Those suffering from vertigo, or
cervical problems should not press
their chin downwards

Bakasana
Crane Pose

Stand straight. Bend forward from the waist resting your hands on the ground under your shoulders and look down. Raise one leg off the floor straight behind you while keeping the heel of the other leg off the ground. Hold the posture for 10–30 seconds.
Repeat with the other leg.

Breathing: **Normal**

Benefits

▶ Strengthens and increases the flexibility of the back
▶ Improves sense of balance
▶ Tones and shapes the hips
▶ Strengthens the neck muscles

Cautions

▶ Those with severe back problems should not practise this
▶ Those with severe vertigo should avoid raising their heads

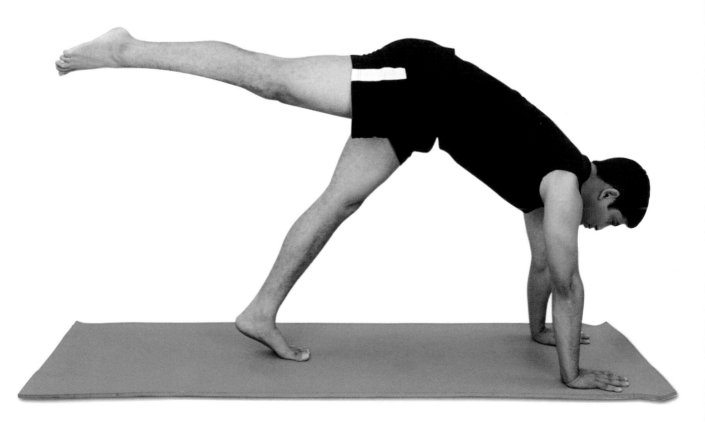

SIDES

These *asanas* work on the latissimus dorci muscles that originate under the armpit and go down to the hips. Practised regularly, they help to remove the excess fat from the sides giving you a V-shaped body.

Ardha Chakrasana
The Half Wheel

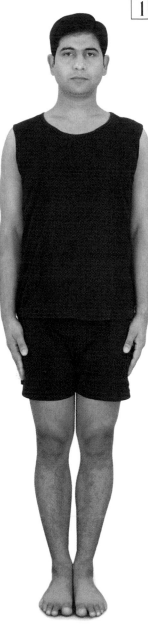

1 Stand straight with your hands at the side of your thighs and look straight in front.

2 Inhale and slowly raise your left hand at right angles to your body.

S I D E S

3
Pull your arm upwards over your
head so that the shoulder touches
the ear. Exhale, bend to the right,
and slide your right hand down
the side of your leg. Tilt your head
sideways and hold this posture for
10–30 seconds.
Repeat on the other side.

Breathing: **Normal**

Benefits

▶ Removes fat from the sides of the
  body
▶ Helps get rid of stiff hip joints
▶ Helps in curing asthma
  (The functional capacity of each lung
  is enhanced when you bend and the
  load of both lungs is taken by one.
  This clears all the blockages of the
  lungs and improves breathing.)

Cautions

▶ Do not bend forwards or backwards
▶ Do not hold your breath

47

Trikonasana
The Triangle

**S
I
D
E
S**

1 Stand with your legs apart. Bend your left arm and place your left hand under the armpit.

2 Bend sideways, exhale slowly and slide your right hand below the right knee. Hold the posture for 10–30 seconds.
Repeat on the other side.

Breathing: **Normal**

Benefits
▶ Helps to remove the fat from the outer sides of the thighs
▶ Actively stretches the waist and passively stretches the upper body
▶ Tones the entire sides of the body

Caution
▶ Those with high blood pressure, vertigo or severe back problems should not practise this

Hasta Kona Trikonasana
The Tilted Triangle

Benefits

▶ Helps remove fat from the waist and trunk

▶ Strengthens the ligaments of the thighs and the muscles of the back

Caution

▶ Those with high blood pressure, vertigo or severe back problems should not practise this

S I D E S

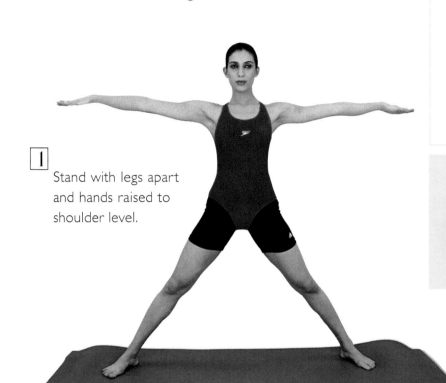

1 Stand with legs apart and hands raised to shoulder level.

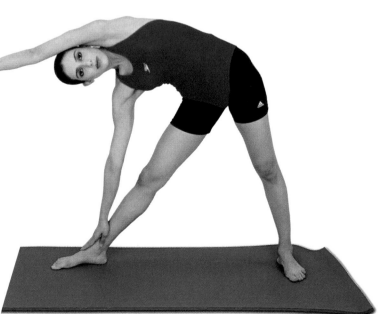

2 Point the right toe outward and raise your left arm above your head. Exhale, and slide the right hand down the leg and bend to the side. Keep the left arm straight, the palm pointing in the same direction as the right foot. Hold for 10–30 seconds. Repeat on the other side.

Breathing: **Normal**

Triyakatadasana
Standing Half Wheel

Benefits

▶ Stretches the arms and the upper sides of the trunk

▶ Improves the flexibility of the spine and the muscles of the back

Stand with legs apart and hands raised above the head. Grip the right wrist with the left hand. Exhale, and bend to the left from the waist. Hold for 10–30 seconds. Inhale and return to upright position. Repeat on the opposite side.

Breathing: Normal

Caution

▶ Those with frozen shoulder or severe back problems should not practise this

S I D E S

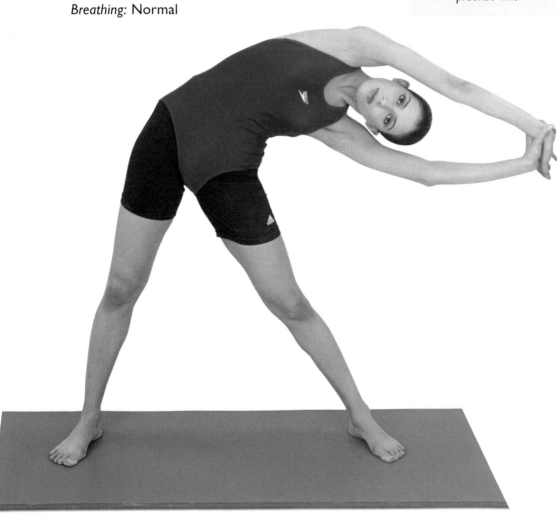

Parigharasana
Sitting Side Stretch

Benefits

▶ Stretches the muscles of the pelvic region, trunk, arms and thighs

▶ Strengthens the back muscles

1 Kneel on the left knee and stretch the right leg out to the side pointing your toes outward.

Cautions

▶ Those with severe back problems should not practise this

▶ Those with knee pain should place a cushion underneath the bent knee

S I D E S

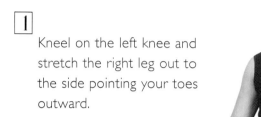

2 Raise the left hand above the head and place the right hand on the hip. Exhale and bend to the right. Hold for 10–30 seconds. Inhale and come back up.
Repeat on the opposite side.

Breathing: **Normal**

Uthitatrikonasana
The Extended Triangle

**S
I
D
E
S**

Spread your feet wide apart. Turn your right foot away at 90 degrees. Raise your hands to shoulder level. Turn your body to the right. Exhaling, place the right hand on the floor outside your right knee. With the left arm reach as far as you can over your right foot. Hold for 10–30 seconds.
Repeat on the other side.

Breathing: **Normal**

Benefits
▶ Helps remove extra fat from the thighs
▶ Tones and massages the pelvic region
▶ Strengthens the arms

Caution
▶ Those with high blood pressure or a stiff neck should not practise this

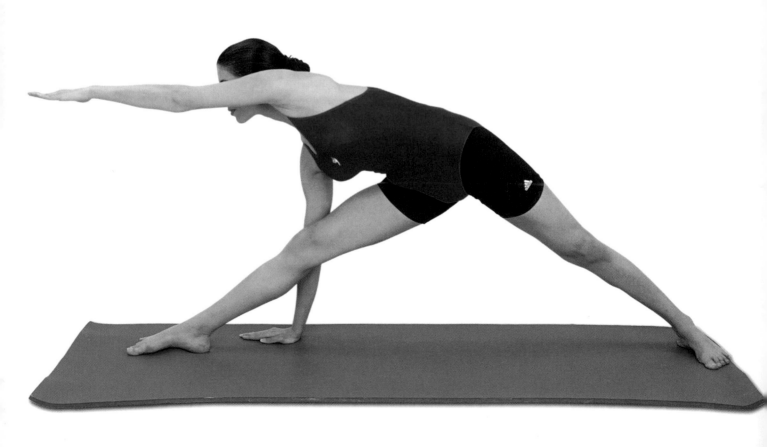

UPPER BODY

These *asanas* work on the arms, chest, shoulders, upper side muscles and neck. Practised regularly, they will strengthen and improve the shape of your upper body and give you a good posture.

Ardhachandrasana
Half Moon Pose

UPPER BODY

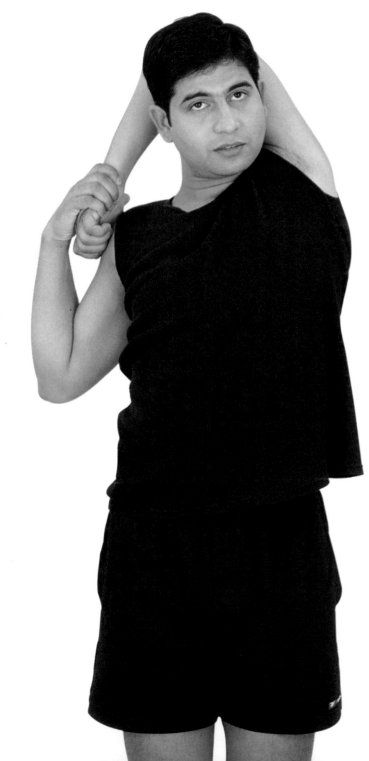

Take the left arm behind the head and hold the left wrist with the right hand. Pull and hold for 10–30 seconds. Repeat on the other side.

Breathing: **Normal**

Benefits

- Increases flexibility of the shoulders
- Tones and shapes the upper back
- Removes stiffness in the neck

Cautions

- Those with frozen shoulder should not practise this
- Those with lower back pain should be careful while practising this

Gomukhasana
Head-of-Cow Pose

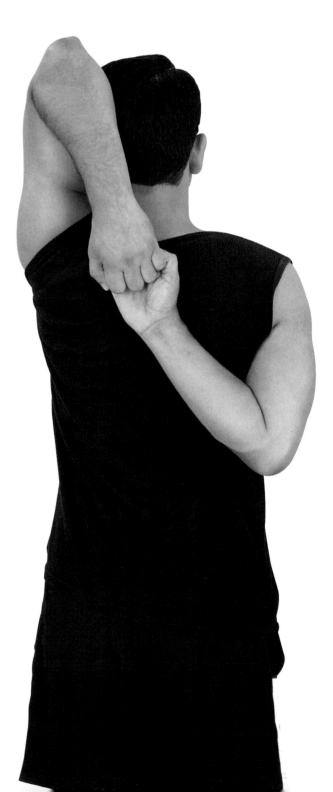

Benefits

▶ Increases the flexibility of the arms and shoulder blades

▶ Opens the chest and improves the respiration

▶ Tones and shapes the back

Caution

▶ Those with frozen shoulder should not practise this

U P P E R B O D Y

Place the left hand behind your shoulders and reaching behind your back with the other hand, interlock the fingers of both hands. Pull and hold for 10–30 seconds.
Interchange the arms and repeat the exercise.

Breathing: **Normal**

Santolanasana
Balancing Pose

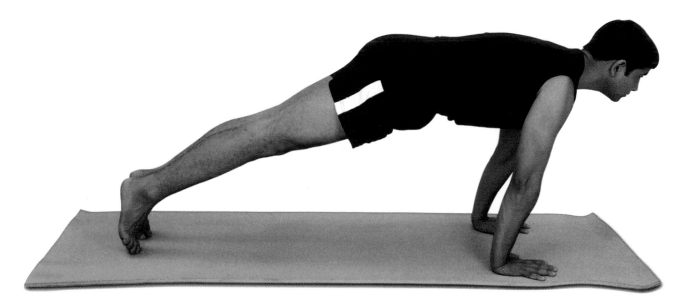

Lie down on your stomach with your hands beside your chest. Raise your body into a push-up position and then move it forward as far as possible keeping your toes in a fixed position. Hold for 10–30 seconds.

Breathing: Normal

Benefits

▶ Strengthens and tones the arms
▶ Strengthens the back and neck
▶ Increases flexibility of the shoulder joints

Caution

▶ Those with severe back problems or a tennis elbow should not practise this

Ek Hastha Santolanasana
One Hand Balancing Pose

Benefits

▶ Strengthens the arms, upper body and back

▶ Improves balance, concentration and will-power

Caution

▶ Those with frozen shoulder or neck problems should be careful while practising this

U P P E R B O D Y

Lie down on your stomach. Raise your body into the push-up position and then place one hand behind your back. Hold for 10–30 seconds.
Repeat with the other arm.

Breathing: **Normal**

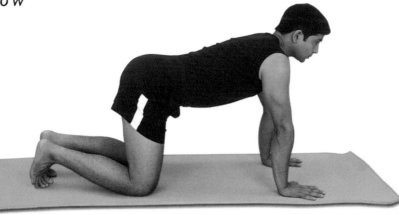

Dwetasana
The Bow

**U
P
P
E
R

B
O
D
Y**

Benefits
▶ Strengthens the elbows and wrists
▶ Strengthens and shapes the upper body

Caution
▶ Those suffering from upper backache or chest pains should not practise this

1 Kneel on the floor and lower your upper body resting on the palms and parallel to the ground.

2 Raise one leg and bring your chest down so that your chin is just above the floor and hold for 10–30 seconds. Repeat with the other leg.

Breathing: Normal

Parsh Konasana
Side Arm Raise

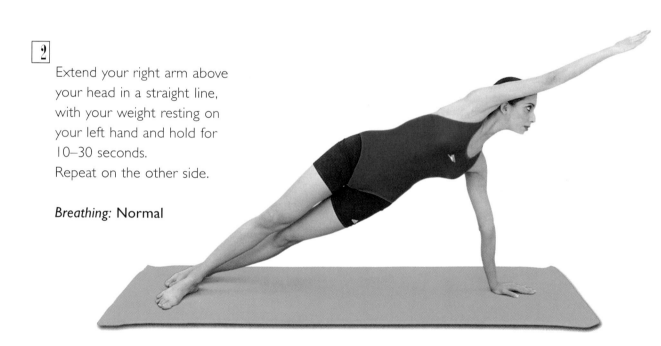

1 Lie down on your stomach. Raise your body into the push-up position. Now turn your entire body to the right keeping one palm on the floor and the other facing the body, with both feet facing the same direction.

2 Extend your right arm above your head in a straight line, with your weight resting on your left hand and hold for 10–30 seconds.
Repeat on the other side.

Breathing: **Normal**

U P P E R   B O D Y

Benefits

▶ Tones the arms and sides of the body
▶ Improves the sense of balance
▶ Strengthens the neck

Caution

▶ Those with back problems or suffering from frozen shoulder should be careful while practising this

Ek Pad Uttana Santolanasana

The Half Bow

Stand straight and bend forwards
placing your palms on the floor some
distance from your feet. Raise one leg
into the air keeping it in a straight line
with your torso. Hold for 10–30
seconds.
Repeat with the other leg.

Breathing: **Normal**

Benefits

▶ Strengthens the arms, shoulders
and wrists
▶ Strengthens the chest muscles
▶ Shapes the upper body

Caution

▶ Those suffering from frozen
shoulder should be careful
while practising this

BACK

These *asanas* work on all the muscles associated with the back, lower, upper and middle. Practised regularly, they will strengthen and keep your back straight, give you a perfect S-curve and a good posture.

Saralhasta Bhujangasana
The Half Cobra

1 Lie flat on your stomach, arms
by your side.

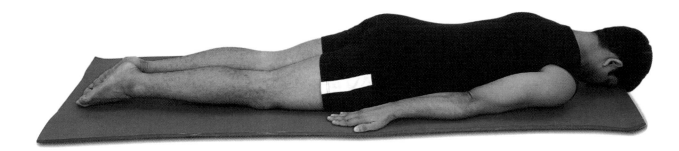

2 Place your hands by your chest,
elbows up, tucked in.

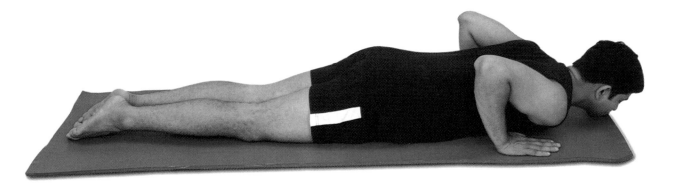

Benefits

▶ Helps to remove stiffness from the chest, shoulders and neck

▶ Stretches the abdominal muscles and helps to remove flab from the abdomen

▶ Alleviates many male urino-genital problems and female gynaecological problems

▶ Alleviates lower back pain by strengthening the muscles of the back

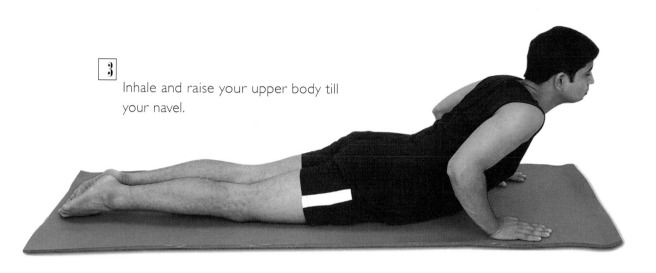

3 Inhale and raise your upper body till your navel.

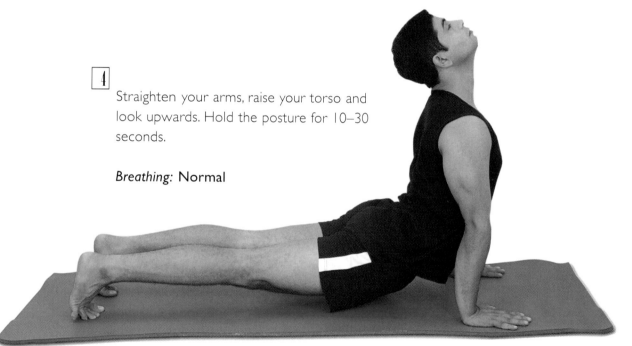

4 Straighten your arms, raise your torso and look upwards. Hold the posture for 10–30 seconds.

Breathing: **Normal**

Cautions

▶ Those who have undergone abdominal surgery or are suffering from hernia or hydrocele should not practise this
▶ Those with severe backache or spinal injury should consult their doctor before attempting this

Marjariariasana
The Cock

Benefits

▶ Improves the flexibility and strength of the back

▶ Removes postural defects like a rounded back

Caution

▶ Practise this gently and slowly and avoid jerks

1 Place your palms and knees on the ground. Inhale and look upwards, curving your back.

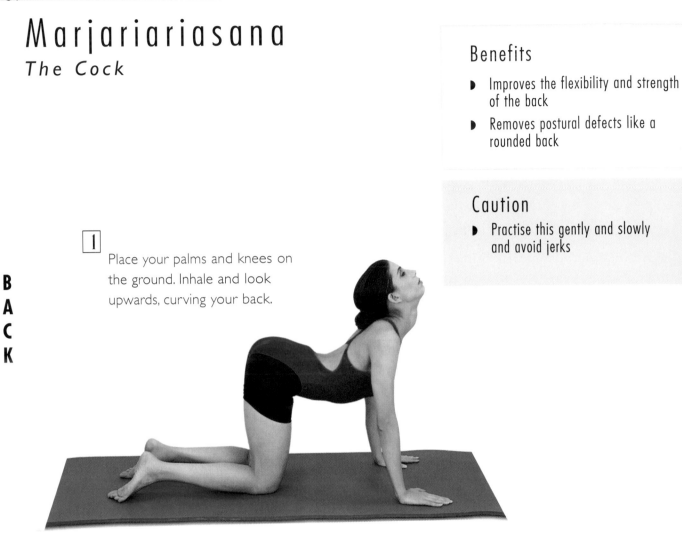

2 Exhale and curve your back inwards and look at your navel. Hold the posture for 10–30 seconds

Breathing: **Normal**

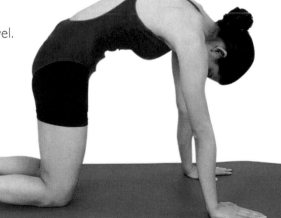

Sahaj Pavanmuktasana
Half Child Pose

1 Lie on your back, arms by your side. Fold the right knee and place the foot close to your hip.

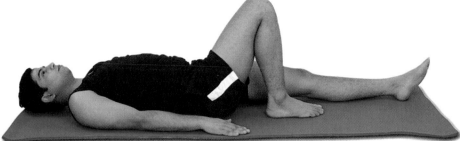

2 Clasp your right knee with your hands. Inhale and bring it close to your chest.

B A C K

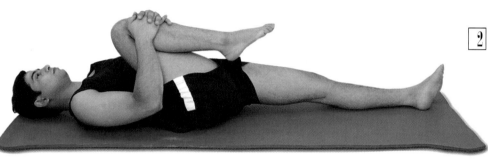

3 Bring your chin to your knee and hold the posture for 10–30 seconds. Repeat with the other leg.

Breathing: Normal

Benefits

- Removes lower backache and stiffness in the lumbar area
- Stretches the hamstring and the hips, removing the extra fat
- Improves flexibility of the hip and knee joints
- Removes unwanted flatulence

Caution

- Those suffering from cervical spondylitis should keep their head on the floor and not raise their chin

Poorna Pavanmuktasana
Child Pose

Benefits

▶ Removes stiffness from the lower back

▶ Removes fat from the hip

▶ Alleviates pain in the knee joint

▶ Removes unwanted flatulence

Cautions

▶ Those suffering from cervical spondylitis should keep their head on the floor and not raise their chin

▶ Those with flatulence should breathe normally in the final posture

Lie down on your back, arms by your sides. Inhale, clasp both your knees with your hands and bring them close to your chest. Raise your chin to touch your knees. Hold this posture for 10–30 seconds.

Breathing: **Normal**

Chakrasana
The Bilsse
The Bridge

1 Lie down on your back. Fold your knees and place your feet near your hips. Place your palms underneath your shoulders with your fingers pointing towards your feet.

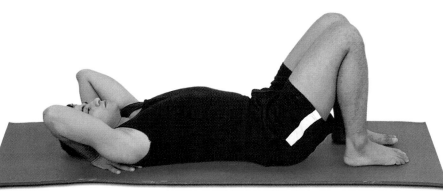

2 Raise your hips.

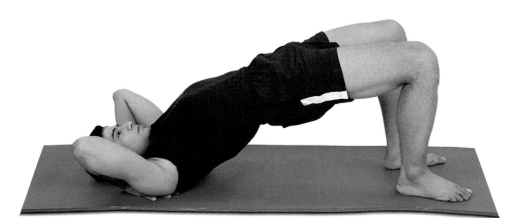

3 Arch your back, shifting your weight onto your hands.

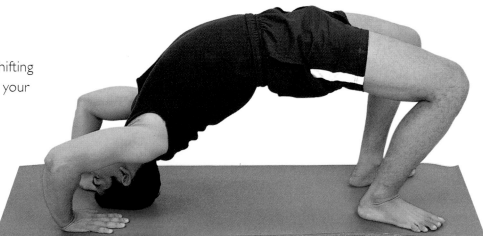

Benefits

▶ Removes fat from the sides of the body
▶ Helps get rid of stiff hip joints
▶ Helps in curing asthma

Cautions

▶ Do not bend forwards and backwards
▶ Do not hold your breath

B
A
C
K

4 Pushing up, raise your head and upper body as far as you can and hold for 10–30 seconds.

Breathing: **Normal**

Merudandasana
The Spinal Twist

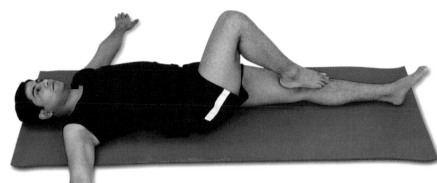

1 Lie down on your back, arms outstretched. Place your right foot on your left knee.

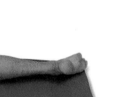

2 Exhale and roll your right knee to the left and look to your right. Press your right knee as close to the floor as possible and hold for 10–30 seconds.
Repeat with the other leg.

Breathing: **Normal**

Benefits

▶ Alleviates stiffness and pain in the upper and mid back and makes it more flexible
▶ Massages the internal organs of the stomach
▶ Stretches the trapeze muscles above the collar bone removing stiffness
▶ Controls sciatica pain

Caution

▶ Those suffering from severe sciatica should consult their doctor before practising this

Dhanurasana

The Arched Bow

B A C K

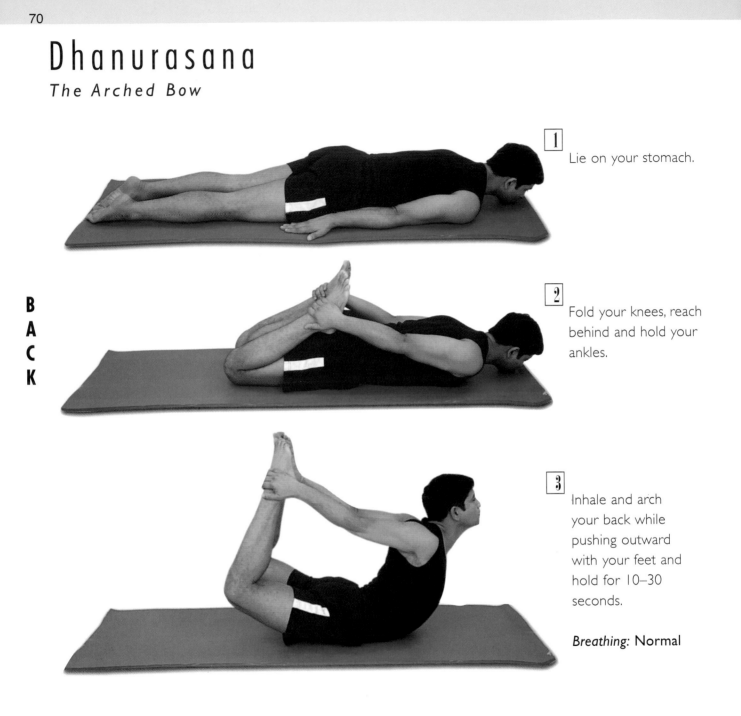

1 Lie on your stomach.

2 Fold your knees, reach behind and hold your ankles.

3 Inhale and arch your back while pushing outward with your feet and hold for 10–30 seconds.

Breathing: Normal

Benefits

- Strengthens the back and abdominal muscles and removes mid backache
- Strengthens the shoulders and arms

Caution

- Those with severe lumbar and cervical pain should not practise this

Viprit Naukasana
The Boat

1 Lie down flat on your stomach with your arms stretched forward.

B A C K

2 Inhale and arch your back, raising your upper body and your legs at the same time and raise your arms upwards. Hold for 10–30 seconds

Breathing: **Normal**

Benefits

▸ Strengthens the entire abdominal area, from the upper to the lower abdomen

Caution

▸ Those with back problems should only practise this when there is no pain

Viprit Ardha Naukasana
Back Leg Stretch

1 Lie down flat on your stomach with your arms stretched forward.

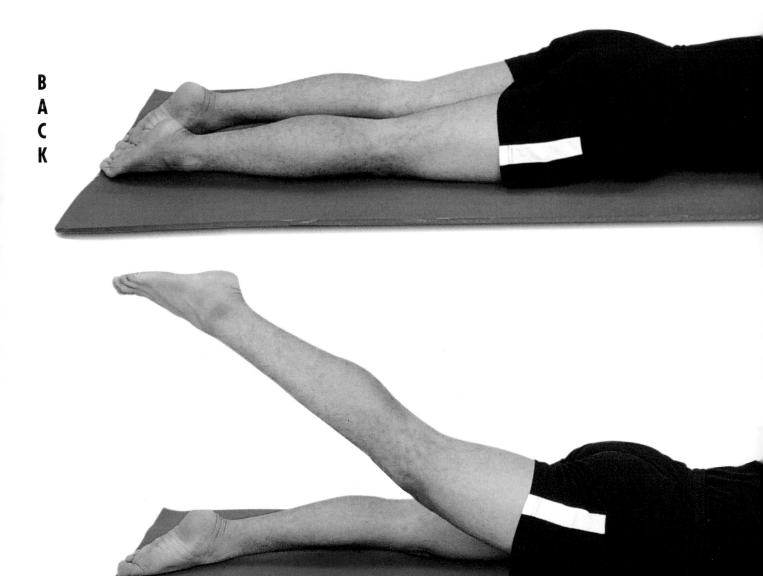

Benefits

▶ Strengthens the back

▶ Cures frozen shoulder if arms are stretched forward slowly

Caution

▶ Those with severe backache should do this very gently

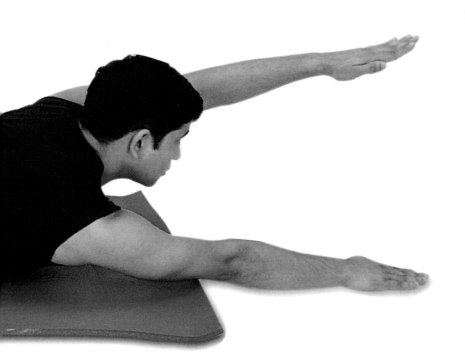

2

Inhale and raise your right leg and your left arm at the same time. Keep your shoulder and ear together when raising your arm. The raised leg should be in the centre of the bodyline. Hold for 10–30 seconds. Repeat on the other side.

Breathing: **Normal**

Dwikonasana
Interlocked Back Hand Raise

Benefits

▶ Removes stiffness from the upper back

▶ Helps to cure cervical spondylitis

▶ Improves the posture of the spine

Cautions

▶ Those with frozen shoulder should raise their hands only as much as possible

▶ Those with vertigo should stop if they feel giddy

1 Stand straight. Reach behind and hold your right wrist with your left hand.

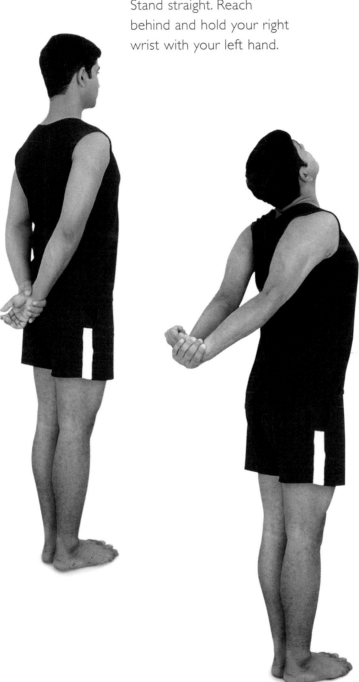

B A C K

2 Inhale, look up and raise your arms upwards. Hold for 10–30 seconds. Interchange your hands and repeat.

Breathing: **Normal**

ABDOMEN

These *asanas* work on the abdominal muscles on the front and sides of your body. Practised regularly, they will give you a well-toned and flat abdomen.

Uthaan Padasana
Half Candle Pose

A B D O M E N

1 Lie flat on your back, arms by your side, palms facing downwards.

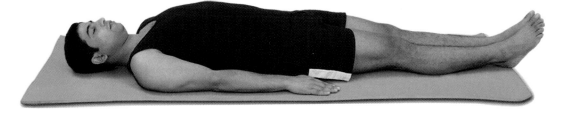

2 Inhale and raise your legs 45 degrees. Hold the posture for 10–30 seconds.

Breathing: Normal

Benefits
▸ Strengthens and massages the abdominal muscles
▸ Improves flexibility of the spine
▸ Tones and strengthens the thighs

Caution
▸ Those with back problems should support the back by placing their hands under their thighs

Ardha Halasana
Supine Leg Raise

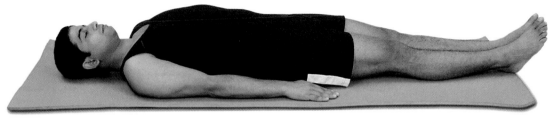

1 Lie flat on your back, arms by your side, palms facing downwards.

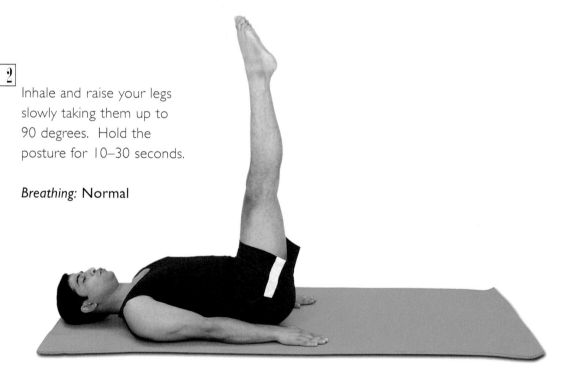

2 Inhale and raise your legs slowly taking them up to 90 degrees. Hold the posture for 10–30 seconds.

Breathing: Normal

A B D O M E N

Benefits

▶ Strengthens and tones the upper abdominal muscles and activates blood circulation
▶ Strengthens the back muscles

Caution

▶ Those with severe back problems and older people with weak muscles should not practise this

Ardha Naukasana
Half Boat Pose

A
B
D
O
M
E
N

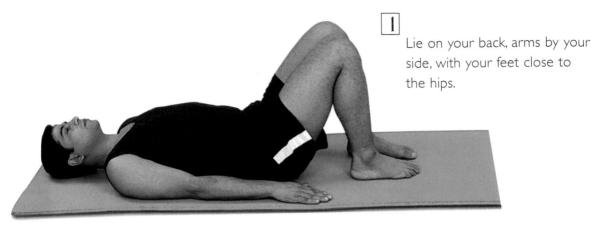

1 Lie on your back, arms by your side, with your feet close to the hips.

2 Inhale, raise your legs parallel to the ground making an angle of 90 degrees. Now exhale and raise your upper body to make a U, with your arms outstretched. Hold the posture for 10–30 seconds.

Breathing: **Normal**

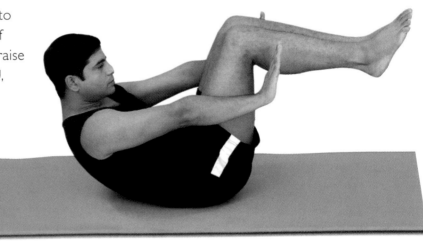

Benefits

▶ Removes excess fat from the abdomen

▶ Tones and strengthens the lower abdomen muscle

▶ Strengthens the back and shoulders

Caution

▶ Those with neck or lower back problems should not practise this

Poorna Naukasana
Complete Boat Pose

1 Lie flat on your back, arms on the thighs and inhale.

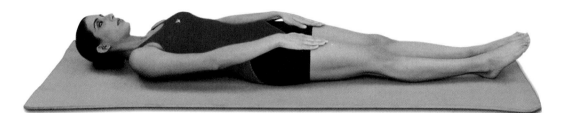

2 Exhale and raise your legs and your upper body 45 degrees above the ground. Stretch your arms straight out towards your toes making a 'boat' shape. Hold the posture for 10–30 seconds.

Breathing: Normal

Benefits

▶ Takes excess weight off your abdomen

▶ Strengthens and tones your middle abdomen

▶ Strengthens the back and thigh muscles

Caution

▶ Those with neck or lower back problems should not practise this

Kati Naukasana

Side Boat Pose

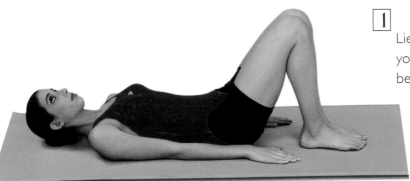

1 Lie flat on your back, arms by your side, with your knees bent. Inhale.

2 Bring your legs up parallel to the ground making an angle of 90 degrees. Exhale, turn your torso sideways and stretch your arms on the other side of your knees. Hold the posture for 10–30 seconds. Repeat on the other side.

Breathing: **Normal**

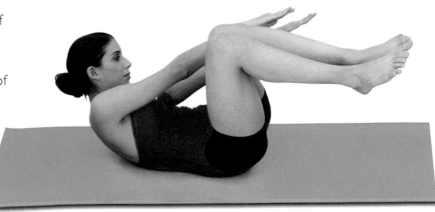

Benefits

- Strengthens and tones the lower abdominal muscles
- Helps remove excess fat from the sides of the abdomen
- Strengthens the thigh, back and shoulder muscles

Cautions

- Those with severe back and neck problems should not practise this
- Those with cervical spondylitis should avoid turning their neck

Duipad Uthaan Kati Naukasana
Raised Boat Pose

1 Lie flat on the back, arms by your side. Inhale, raise your legs and your upper body 60 degrees above the ground, with your arms stretched out towards the knees.

A B D O M E N

2 Exhale and turn your torso sideways bringing your arms by the side of your thighs and look towards your hands. Hold the posture for 10–30 seconds.

Breathing: **Normal.**

Benefits

▶ Strengthens and tones the middle abdomen
▶ Strengthens the back muscles
▶ Reduces fat from the sides of the abdomen

Cautions

▶ Those with severe backache should not practise this
▶ Those with cervical spondylitis should avoid turning their neck

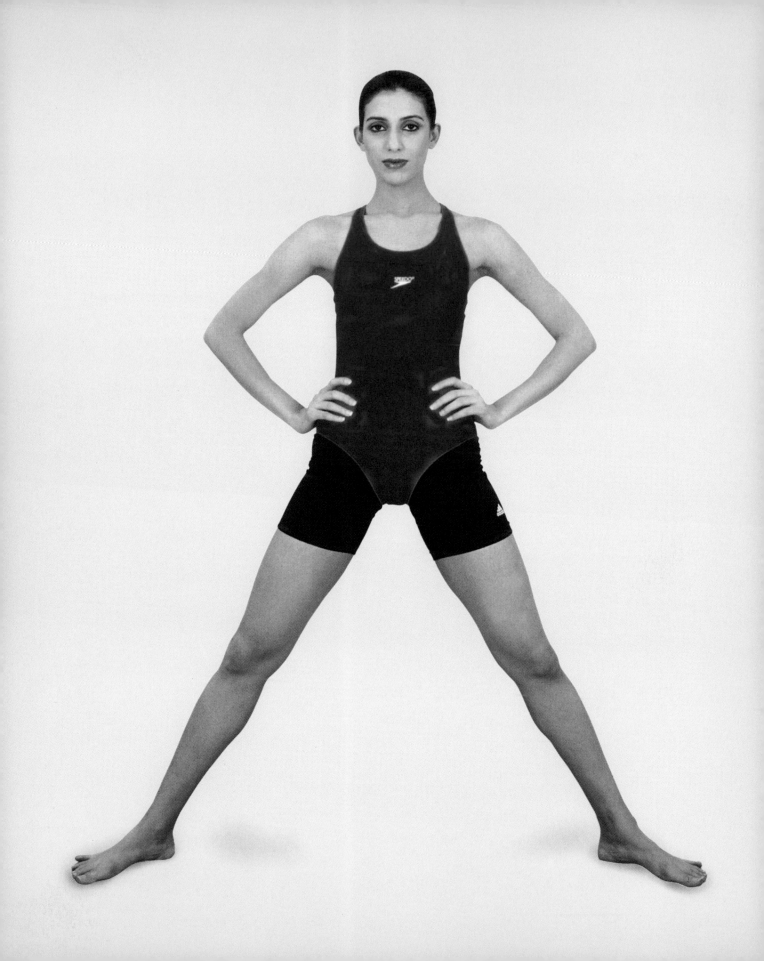

INVERTED POSTURES

These *asanas* increase the flow of blood to your head and face and shift your awareness from the feet to the head. Practised regularly, they bring lustre to your face, give your skin a nice texture and make your eyes clear and bright.

Vipritkarnimudra
Half Shoulderstand

|1|

Lie on your back with your hands by your side. Slowly raise both your legs.

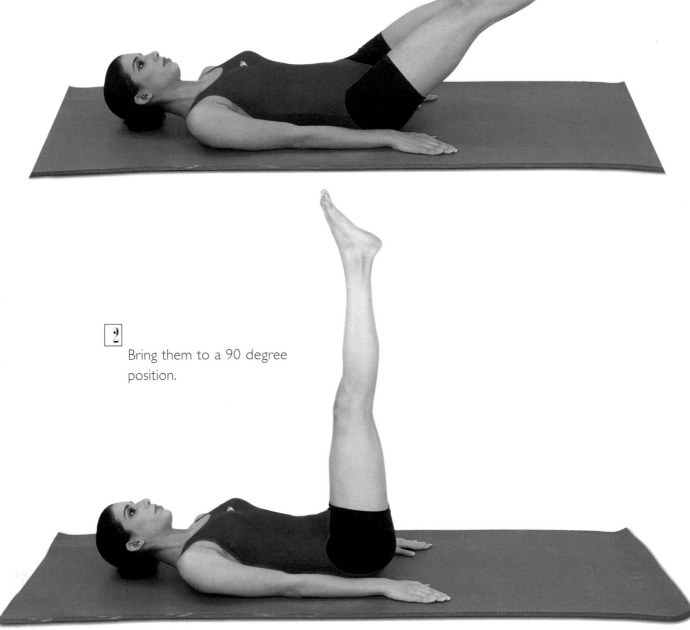

|2|

Bring them to a 90 degree position.

Benefits

▶ Improves the blood circulation to the face and upper part of the body

▶ Improves the glow on the face and helps in removing pimples, patches and pigmentation

▶ Helps in healthy hair growth, reduces immature graying of hair and even hair loss

▶ Clears the blockages in the arteries

Caution

▶ Those suffering from hernia, high blood pressure or spinal injury should not practise this

3

Lift your hips and support them with your hands and hold for 10–30 seconds.

Breathing: Normal

INVERTED POSTURES

Saravangasana
Shoulderstand

I
N
V
E
R
T
E
D

P
O
S
T
U
R
E
S

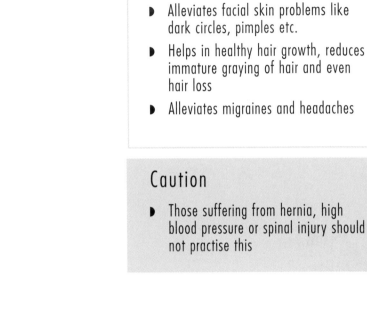

Benefits

▶ Improves the blood flow to the head and enhances all mental faculties

▶ Alleviates facial skin problems like dark circles, pimples etc.

▶ Helps in healthy hair growth, reduces immature graying of hair and even hair loss

▶ Alleviates migraines and headaches

Caution

▶ Those suffering from hernia, high blood pressure or spinal injury should not practise this

Lie on your back with your hands by your side. Slowly raise both your legs. Bring them to a 90 degree position. Lift your hips and back keeping your legs straight with your hands supporting your back. Your weight should rest on your shoulders and elbows. Hold for 10–30 seconds.

Breathing: **Normal**

Halasana
The Plough

1 Lie on your back with your hands by your side. Slowly raise both your legs. Bring them over your head parallel to the ground.

Benefits

▶ Improves the flexibility of the back

▶ Increases the flow of blood to the face, improves the skin texture and removes dark circles under the eyes

▶ Clears the blockages of important internal vital plexus of the body such as the heart and throat

Caution

▶ Those suffering from severe backache, high blood pressure or vertigo should not practise this

2 Lower your legs and touch your toes to the floor.

3 Interlock your hands at the top of your head, resting your weight on your shoulders and toes and hold for 10–30 seconds.

Breathing: Normal

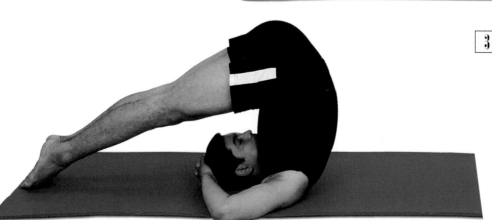

INVERTED POSTURES

Sharnagatmudra
Surrender Pose

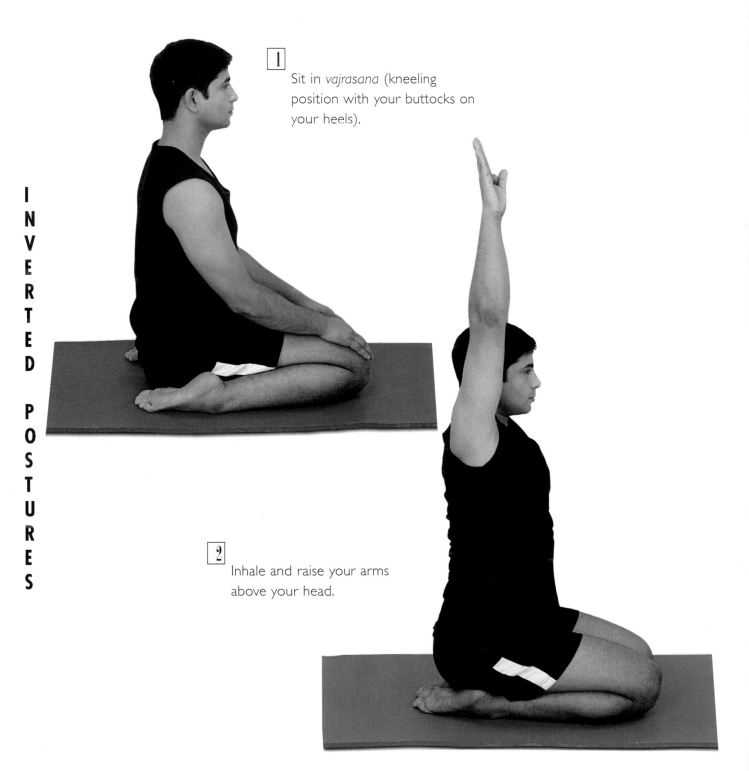

1 Sit in *vajrasana* (kneeling position with your buttocks on your heels).

2 Inhale and raise your arms above your head.

Benefits

▶ Improves flexibility of the back

▶ Helps to relax and relieves stress

▶ Improves skin texture of the face

▶ Strengthens and improves the flexibility of the ankle and knee joints

Caution

▶ Those suffering from backache or severe arthritis of the knee joints should not practise this

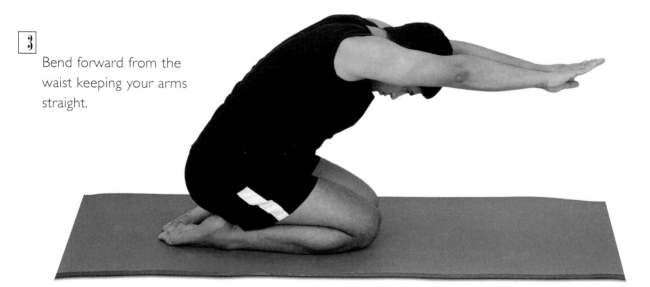

3 Bend forward from the waist keeping your arms straight.

4 With your chest against your knees, touch your head to the floor with your arms extended in front of you and hold for 10–30 seconds.

Breathing: Normal

INVERTED POSTURES

Sirshasana 1
Headstand

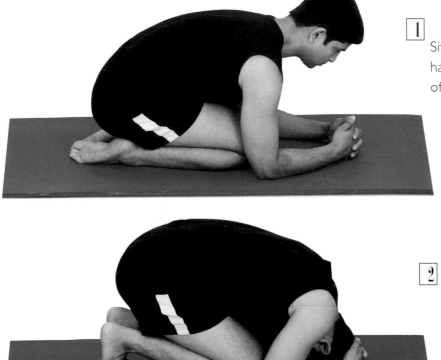

1 Sit in *vajrasana*, interlock your hands and place them in front of you on the floor.

2 Rest the crown of your head in the hollow of your palms, with the top of your forehead resting on the floor.

3 Now raise your hips by straightening your legs. Move your feet towards your head until your torso is vertical.

4 Let your weight rest on your elbows and head and with knees bent raise your feet slowly in the air.

Benefits

- Improves the blood flow to the head and enhances all mental faculties
- Alleviates all facial skin problems such as dark circles, pimples etc.
- Helps in healthy hair growth, reduces immature graying of hair and even hair loss
- Alleviates migraines and headaches
- Strengthens the neck muscles
- Improves the sense of balance

Cautions

- Those suffering from high blood pressure should not practise this
- This should not be practised alone until it has been mastered

5 When you maintain your balance, extend your feet straight into the air and hold for 10–30 seconds.

Breathing: Normal

Bak Sirshasana 2
Open Leg Headstand

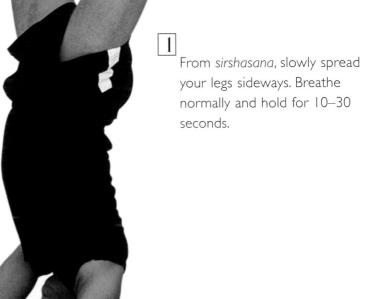

1 From *sirshasana*, slowly spread your legs sideways. Breathe normally and hold for 10–30 seconds.

Benefits

▶ In addition to the benefits of *sirshasana*, this improves the flexibility of the groin area

Cautions

▶ Those suffering from high blood pressure should not practise this

▶ This should not be practised alone until it has been mastered

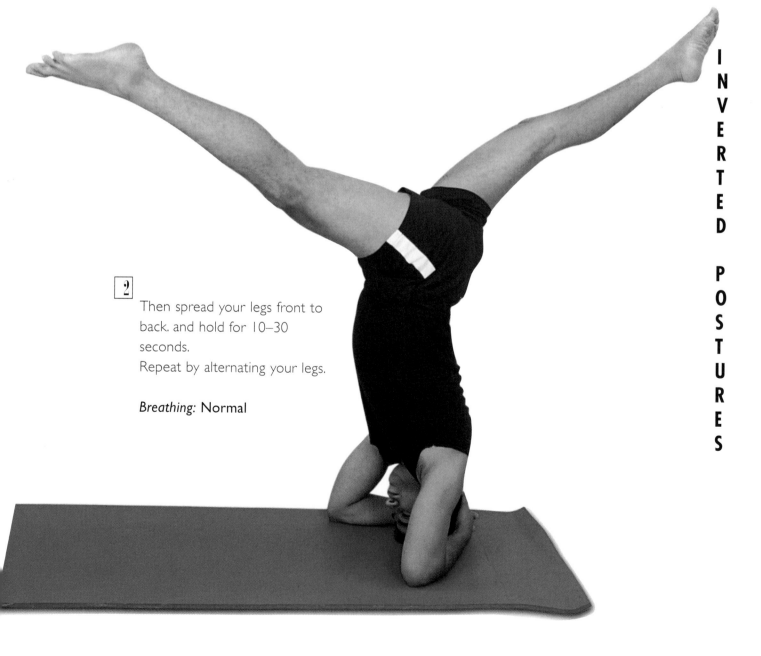

2
Then spread your legs front to back. and hold for 10–30 seconds.
Repeat by alternating your legs.

Breathing: Normal

INVERTED POSTURES

Padma Sirshasana 3
Lotus Headstand

1 From *sirshasana*, fold your legs as in the lotus pose or *padmasana* (see page 96).

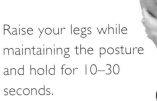

Benefits

- In addition to the benefits of *sirshasana*, it improves your coordination and balance
- Increases blood circulation in the pelvic region
- Alleviates disorders of the reproductive system

Cautions

- Those suffering from high blood pressure should not practise this
- This should not be practised alone until it has been mastered

2 Raise your legs while maintaining the posture and hold for 10–30 seconds.

Breathing: Normal

MEDITATIVE POSTURES

These *asanas* are practised to centre oneself and reach a meditative state, which is the real aim of yoga. Of the 840,000 postures, the sole aim is to be able to stay in one of these meditative postures for an extended period of time.

Padmasana
Lotus Pose

1 Sit comfortably with your knees bent. Place your right foot on the left thigh.

Benefits
▶ Removes stiffness from the knee joints
▶ Improves postural defects of the spine

Caution
▶ Those who have undergone knee or spinal surgery or suffer from severe arthritis should not practise this

2 Holding the toe of the left foot, place it on top of the right thigh.

3 Pull both heels as close as possible to the navel region and try to press both the knees on the floor. Put your hands on your knees touching the tips of the thumbs and forefingers. Keep your back straight and breathe normally.

Breathing: **Normal**

Vajrasana
Diamond Pose

Benefits

- Hastens the digestion of food and can be practised soon after a meal
- Increases the flexibility of the ankle joints
- Improves the posture
- Beneficial for the reproductive organs

Caution

- Those who have undergone knee or spinal surgery or suffer from severe arthritis should not practise this

1 Sit down in the long sitting position with your legs straight in front of you and hands by your side.

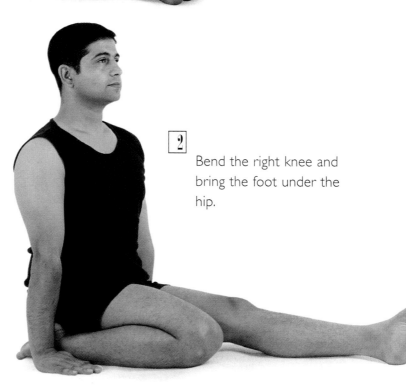

2 Bend the right knee and bring the foot under the hip.

M E D I T A T I V E   P O S T U R E S

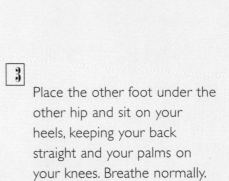

3 Place the other foot under the other hip and sit on your heels, keeping your back straight and your palms on your knees. Breathe normally.

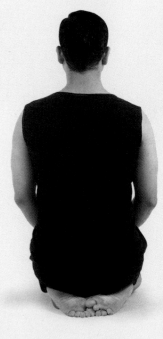

4 The toes should touch each other and the heels should be turned outward making a V.

Breathing: **Normal**

Sukhasana
Easy Pose

Benefits

▶ Easier for those unable to sit in the other meditative postures

▶ Relaxes and balances the whole body

Caution

▶ Avoid sitting in this posture for a long time as you might develop a backache

MEDITATIVE POSTURES

1 Sit with your left leg stretched out and bend your right leg so that your right foot rests between the left thigh and calf muscles.

2 Fold your left leg, bringing the left foot underneath the right thigh.

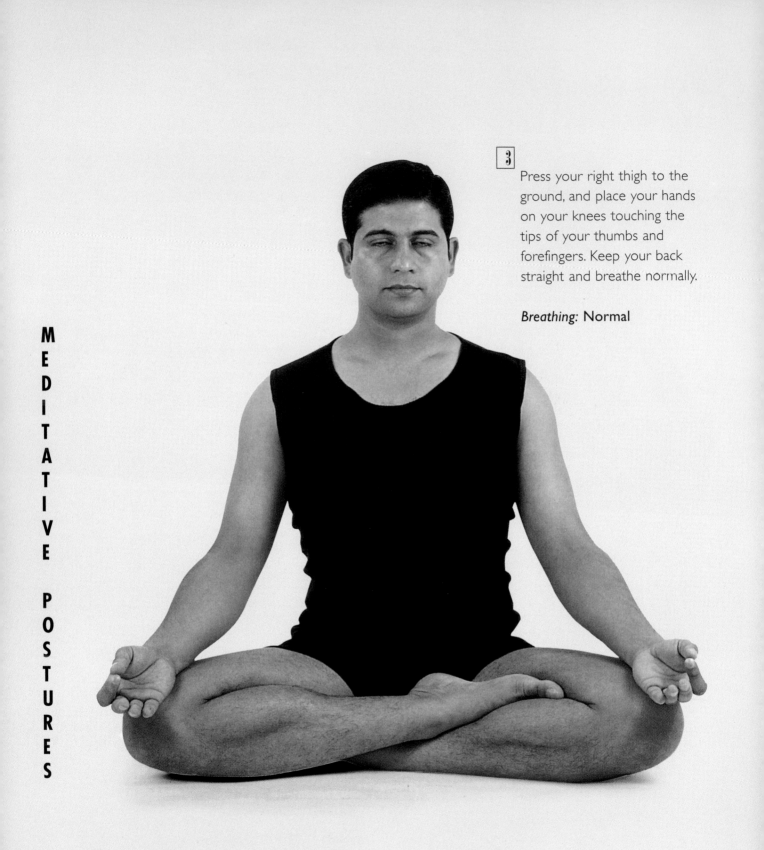

3 Press your right thigh to the ground, and place your hands on your knees touching the tips of your thumbs and forefingers. Keep your back straight and breathe normally.

Breathing: **Normal**

5
Pranayama
(Breath Regulation and Control)

Pranayama is a technique to control breathing which is the link between the mind and the body. *Pranayama* helps to control the mind and increases awareness of oneself without distraction from the thoughts that constantly bombard our minds. It calms the mind by concentrating on one's breathing and ultimately going beyond breathing.

Breath Control

Pranayama decreases the pace of breathing and if practised regularly, can extend one's life. For example, a normal person takes 12–16 breaths per minute. When we sleep we take 30 breaths per minute and 45–60 breaths per minute when we get angry. When we do yoga or *pranayama*, we take one or two per minute. And according to yoga, age equals the number of breaths. Therefore, by practising *pranayama* we can decrease the breath rate and therefore increase our age.

There are three parts of *pranayama: purak* (controlled inhalation), *kumbhak* (retention) and *rechak* (controlled exhalation). *Kumbhak* is the most important aspect of *pranayama* and it is further sub-divided into three parts.

Antar kumbhak – inhaling and stopping the breath.

Wahiyah kumbhak – exhaling and stopping the breath.

Kevala kumbhak – surviving without air for a period of time. This is a gift of practice of *pranayama*, when the whole breathing system ceases and man can still survive.

How *Pranayama* Works

There are two kinds of respiration taking place in our body – external and internal. External respiration is the act of inhaling and exhaling air with the lungs. Internal respiration is the process by which oxygen from the air is transferred to the blood, and carbon dioxide from the blood is sent back into the air. When we inhale, air through the nostrils reaches the lungs via the trachea and small alveola sacs in the lungs swell up like balloons. Each alveola sac is surrounded by blood vessels through which the carbon dioxide and oxygen are exchanged. In *pranayama* when we inhale and hold our breath, we allow enough time for the haemoglobin (Hb) in the blood, to react with the oxygen, forming oxyhaemoglobin, which enriches and energises the whole body ($Hb + O_2 = HbO_2$). *Pranayama* therefore is also the art of revitalising the whole system.

The ideal ratio of *purak* (inhalation), *kumbhak* (retention) and *rechak* (exhalation) is 1:4 and 4:2. But initially, one should not hold the breath for four times the inhalation. One should start with a ratio of 1:2:2. After a month, one can move up to 1:3:2. And after three months one can move up to a ratio of 1:4:2. For example, one should start with inhaling for 5 seconds, retaining the breath for 10 seconds and exhaling for 10 seconds. Then one should inhale, retain and exhale in the ratio of 5 seconds: 15 seconds: 10 seconds. Finally one should be able to inhale, retain and exhale in the ratio of 5 seconds: 20 seconds: 10 seconds.

Sheetli Pranayama
Rolled-tongue Breathing

This *pranayama* is practised to lower the temperature of the body and also to reduce anxiety and stress.

TECHNIQUE

Sit in *padmasana* or *sukhasana* with your back straight and eyes preferably closed. Roll your tongue as shown in the picture and slowly inhale through the hole made by the tongue. Count to 5 while inhaling. Press your chin down on your neck, hold your breath and count to 10. Raise your chin, exhale slowly through the nostrils and count to 10.

CYCLE

Repeat this at least 15 times. As you become more comfortable, you can do this for as long as one hour. If you feel very cold then stop it immediately.

This should not be practised in cold weather.

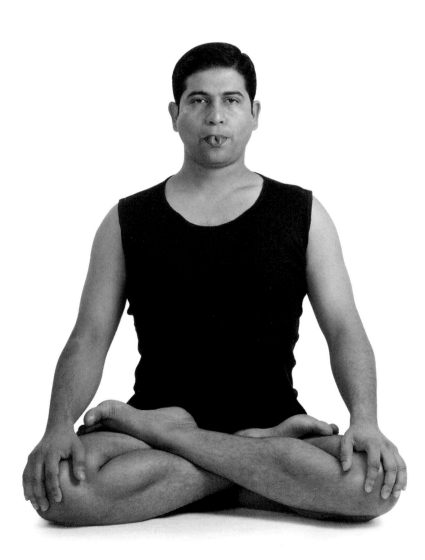

Benefits

▶ Cools the body by lowering the temperature
▶ Reduces anxiety and stress

Caution

▶ Those with high blood pressure and respiratory problems should not practise this

Sheetkari Pranayama
Square-lip Breathing

This *pranayama* is for those who cannot roll their tongue as in *Sheetli pranayama*.

TECHNIQUE

Sit in *padmasana* or *sukhasana* with your back straight and eyes preferably closed. Make a square shape with your lips showing your teeth. Count to 5 while inhaling. Press your chin down on your neck. Hold your breath and count to 10. Raise your chin, exhale slowly through the nostrils and count to 10.

CYCLE

Repeat this at least 15 times. As you become more comfortable, you can do this for as long as one hour. If you feel very cold then stop it immediately.

This should not be practised in cold weather.

Benefits

▶ Cools the body by lowering the temperature.
▶ Reduces anxiety and stress

Cautions

▶ Those with high blood pressure and respiratory problems should not practise this
▶ Stop if there is irritation in the throat

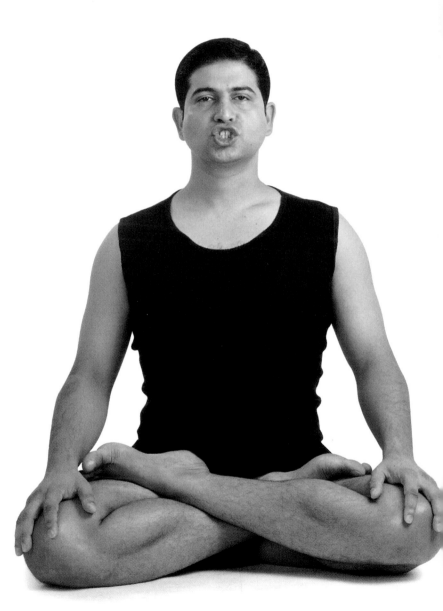

Sahaj Pranayama
Easy Breathing

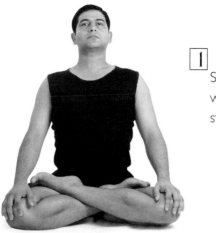

1 Sit in *padmasana* with your back straight.

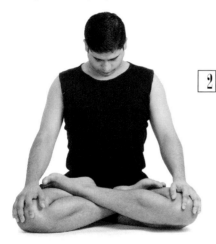

2 Press your chin down on your neck, inhale deeply, and hold your breath.

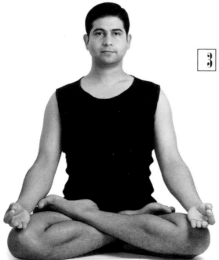

3 Raise your chin and exhale through the mouth. Repeat this 15 times

Benefits

▶ Increases the body temperature, burns calories and reduces weight
▶ Reduces anxiety and stress

Caution

▶ Those with cervical spondylitis should keep their chin up and not press it downwards

Anulom-Vilom Pranayama
Alternate Nostril Breathing

1 Sit in *padmasana* or *sukhasana*, folding the forefinger and middle finger of your right hand.

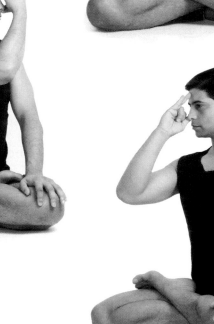

2 Placing your thumb in between your eyebrows, and pressing your ring finger on the left nostril, breathe in through the right nostril. Hold your breath.

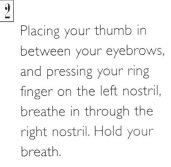

Benefits

- Increases the supply of oxygen to the blood and purifies it by expelling the toxins
- Increases concentration, and simultaneously reduces stress

Caution

- Those with high blood pressure or heart problems should not hold their breath

3 Reverse positions by placing your ring finger between your eyebrows and press your right nostril with your thumb. Exhale through the left nostril. Now inhale through the left nostril and hold. Reverse the position of your fingers as in Step 2 and exhale through the right nostril.
Repeat this cycle 12 times.

Kriyas
(Purification Techniques)

Kriyas, one of the most important aspects of *bahirang* yoga rid the body of all toxins. Environmental pollution, adulteration of food and increased stress levels lead to increased toxins in the body and a strained internal system. These yogic *kriyas* rid our bodies of all the toxins and strengthen the 72,000 *nadis*, which are the channels of energy in our body, forming a kind of electrical circuit system. Sickness is largely due to a problem in this electrical circuit. Of all these *nadis* there are three which regulate all the rest: *ida* (which runs from left nostril), *pingla* (which runs from the right nostril) and *sushmna* (which runs in the cerebro-spinal fluid in the centre of the spine).

Agnisar Kriya
Activating Digestive Fire

1 Stand straight with feet
shoulder width apart. Lower
your body and place your
hands on your thighs, palms
inward.

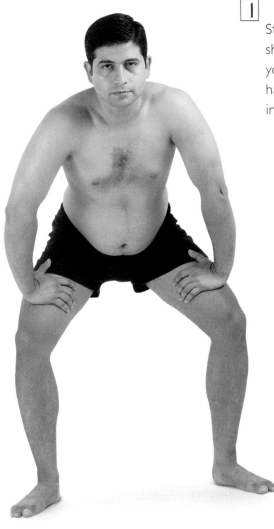

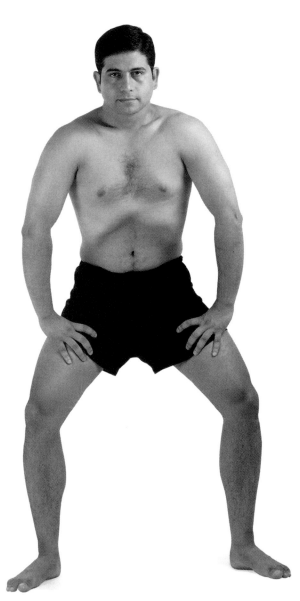

2 Exhale deeply through your
mouth. Holding your breath,
pull your abdominal muscles in.

3

Continue to hold your breath, push your abdominal muscles out and pull them in again. Repeat this cycle 10–70 times.

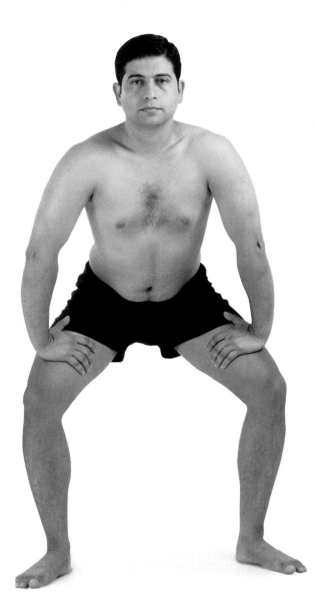

Benefits

▶ Activates the peristaltic movement in the stomach, resulting in better digestion and excretion

▶ Strengthens the abdominal muscles and removes fat from the abdominal area

Cautions

▶ Be careful not to inhale as it might cause stomach problems

▶ Those with a low backache should avoid bending forward

Kapalbhati is the art of exhaling actively and inhaling passively.

TECHNIQUE

Sit in *vajrasana*, or *padmasana*. Place hands on the knees, back upright, eyes looking straight ahead. Exhale forcefully through the nose, and push the stomach inward. Relax the stomach and inhale bringing it back to its original position.

Practise this with 50 exhalations at a stretch, then increase to 100. Subsequently, perform this for 2 minutes continuously and increase the duration to 10 minutes.

Kapalbhati Kriya
Frontal Brain Cleansing Breath

Benefits

▶ Increases the metabolic rate and reduces fat

▶ Improves cardio-respiratory endurance and builds stamina

▶ Activates the peristaltic movement in the stomach, resulting in better digestion and excretion

▶ Helps to cure sinus, migraine and hypertension

▶ Revitalises the system

Caution

▶ Those suffering from high blood pressure, gynaecological problems, stomach ailments or who have undergone recent surgery should consult their doctor before practising this

Dhokan Kriya
Respiratory System Cleansing

Benefits

- Increases the metabolic rate and reduces fat
- Improves cardio-respiratory endurance and builds stamina
- Activates the peristaltic movement in the stomach, resulting in better digestion and excretion
- Strengthens facial muscles and removes wrinkles and laugh lines

Caution

- Those suffering from high blood pressure, gynaecological problems, stomach ailments or who have undergone recent surgery should consult their doctor before practising this

TECHNIQUE

Sit in *vajrasana*, or *padmasana*. Place hands on the knees, back upright, eyes looking straight ahead. Exhale forcefully through the mouth, and push the stomach inward. Relax the stomach and inhale bringing it back to its original position.

Practise this with 50 exhalations at a stretch, then increase to 100. Subsequently, perform this for 2 minutes continuously and increase the duration to 10 minutes.

112

Tratak Kriya
Steady Gazing

Benefits

▸ Clears and brightens the eyes
▸ Improves concentration and ability to focus
▸ Relieves insomnia, depression and stress

Caution

▸ Those with eye problems should not practise this

TECHNIQUE

Place a lighted candle at arms length on a table in front of you at eye level. Sit in any meditative *asana* with your back straight. Close your eyes and relax the body. Then open your eyes and gaze steadily at the tip of the wick. Try not to blink or move your eyeballs. When the eyes get tired after a few minutes, close them and focus on the after image of the candle. After a minute, open your eyes and continue to gaze at the flame. Repeat this 2–3 times. Practise for a total of 2 minutes, slowly going up to 10 minutes at the maximum. Make sure there is no wind and the flame is steady.

Bandhas
(Restoring Hormonal Balance)

Bandhas are neuromuscular locks performed to increase the endocrine (glandular) secretions in our body. Our moods are determined by the levels of hormones in our body. Yogis talk about *ananda maya chitta*, a relaxed and happy state of mind. *Bandhas* are one of those tools that restore the hormonal balance in the body making you happy and relaxed throughout the day.

Jalandhar Bandha
Throat Lock

1 Sit in *padmasana* or *vajrasana*. Inhale deeply, fill your lungs with air, keep your chest high and hold your breath.

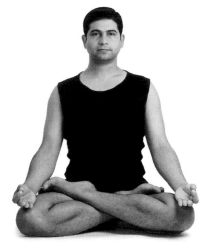

2 Then slowly bend your chin down and press it hard on your neck. Hold your breath for 30 seconds to one minute.

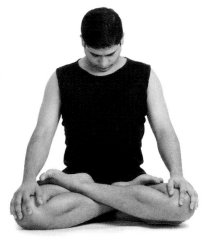

3 Continue to hold your breath and raise your chin, straightening your neck. Exhale through your nostrils. Repeat up to 3 times

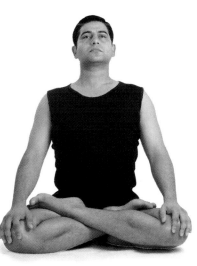

Benefits

▶ Helps in controlling thyroid diseases by increasing the amount of thyroxine produced

▶ Affects the fat deposition in the body by directing the flow of blood to the heart

Caution

▶ Those suffering from cervical spondylitis or with high thyroxine levels should not practise this

Udyan Bandha
Abdominal Lock

1

Stand straight with feet shoulder width apart. Lower your body and place your hands on your thighs, palms inwards. Then exhale deeply through your mouth.

2

Holding your breath, pull your abdominal muscles in and suck in your stomach to create a hollow space. Hold for as long as possible. Stand upright and then inhale. Repeat 2–3 times.

Benefits

- Strengthens the lower abdominal muscles, the excretory system and the glands in the abdominal area
- Alleviates several gynaecological problems
- Helpful for those with asthma, bronchitis, and prostrate problems

Caution

- Those with heart disease or high blood pressure and pregnant women should not practise this

Mool Bandha
Root Lock

TECHNIQUE:

Sit in *padmasana* or *sukhasana*. Exhale deeply through your mouth and hold your breath.

Close your anal space and pull it upward. Pull all your lower abdominal organs and muscles upward and hold as long as possible.

Slowly release the lower abdominal organs. Inhale and relax your body. Bring your breathing back to its normal state.

Repeat up to 3 times.

Benefits

▶ Strengthens the lower abdominal muscles, the excretory system and the glands in the abdominal area

▶ Alleviates several gynaecological problems

▶ Helpful for those with asthma, bronchitis, and prostrate problems

Caution

▶ Those with heart disease or high blood pressure and pregnant women should not practise this

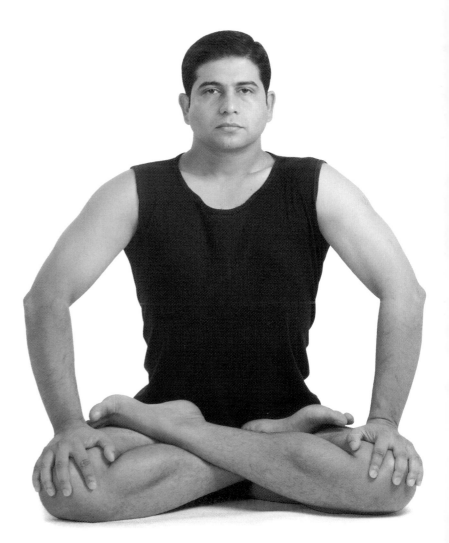

Meditation for
Union of Body and Mind

Meditation, according to yoga, happens when the body reaches an amazing degree of maturity after great *tapas* (effort), which includes its physical and mental reconditioning through all aspects of external yoga – *asana*, *pranayama*, *kriya*, *bandha*. Religions talk about different skills of meditation but yoga takes a much deeper look and regards meditation as a beautifully organised practical system that takes you to oneness of the body and mind. The body put through the rigours of hard *sadhana*, through the practice of *asanas*, can be compared to raw gold which goes through fire to prove its purity. The gold is then beaten and moulded into jewellery by the goldsmith. Yoga acts in much the same way. It prepares the body and the mind and takes one to a stage of complete fitness. Enlightenment – a state where a person is in a state of constant awareness and meditation – cannot happen to a physically unfit, stiff or diseased person.

118

Meditation – Living in the Present

Patanjali in the first sutra says, *Atha Yoga Anushasanam*, which means – now, the discipline of yoga. Now, simply means moving inward. Yoga aims at making a person live in the now. A yogi's aim is to kill the past. Insecurity, fear, possession, anger, selfishness, worry, tension, pain, happiness, agony – all these have to merge in the present. Yoga is not a philosophy, it is a practice, which means that one is actually doing something in the present. The more one practises yoga, the more the present looks real. And if one can be wholly in the present, the whole mystery of man can be realised in a fraction of a second. So meditation is not an explanation, or an achievement. It is a state of living completely in the present, where there is no you. In another words, it is the movement from *you* to *no you*.

Life as Meditation

Yoga is a practice. It has no beliefs or laws. It is pure action. Yoga believes two factors are required for enlightenment – *abhyaas* and *vairagya*. *Abhyaas* means practice. And *vairagya* means attachment inward. Not detachment from outside. Meditation can happen to anyone practising yoga at any stage. This is why yoga never teaches skills of meditation. It talks about the skill of life itself. The goal of yoga is to make every aspect of life meditative in nature.

How Meditation Happens

In order to meditate there must be a release of energy. This can happen only by breakage, and the practice of yoga breaks the body, the mind, the belief system and everything that comes in the way of silence. It simply creates situations to help one try to go beyond oneself. But this is not meditation. It is simply an effort towards meditation. One can start meditating by simply understanding that when your eyes are open you drain energy and when your eyes are closed you divert the energy inside and break the barriers of silence that initially come to you as thoughts. But sooner or later you will get periods of silence in between. Keep expanding them. However, don't create a fight between the silences and your thoughts. Let it happen naturally or else you will end up practising thoughtlessness, which is just a trick of the mind. In these phases of silence you will start moving into a tunnel inside which a man walks when he dies. The day you know this tunnel, the fear of death will leave you and this is what the final goal of meditation is. To know your death before you die.

The candle in *tratak kriya* is used to increase awareness and calm the mind making it more receptive to meditation.

Chanting can be practised with the aid of a *mala* (rosary) which helps to clean the mind and brings you closer to a state of meditation.

The staircase of *samadhi* starts from *sabeej*, (an effort towards silence), where one is still there. This eventually leads to *nirbeej*, where just the awareness remains. The day even awareness disappears, one enters *dharamamega samadhi*. Don't ask anyone what there is beyond this tunnel. You might understand it as a concept and create it with your mind as a mind game, missing out on the real experience. So forget about *chakras* (plexus), *kundalini* (latent energy), *moksha* (salvation), and enlightenment. Just sit down with your eyes closed and nature will reveal the rest to you. In your practice you may only need a master to guide you along and let you know when you have trapped yourself in a mind game.

Principles to Live by

Meditation is not a skill to be practised or learnt. It is the art of expanding one's conscious body that might happen in a second if one is ready. You cannot force meditation to happen, but by practising yoga and following these guiding principles, you can create that readiness in yourself.

1 Accept that the unknown is not in your control so don't try to understand it or have a mastery over it. Just surrender to the unknown. If you have fears and insecurities, accept them and also accept that you are solely responsible for all your pains as you are for your happiness in life.

2 Move towards a non-judgemental state. Yoga talks about constant awareness – a state of complete alertness which can be described thus: when you are very quiet, even a drop falling in a bucket of water, will make a sound. If you judge the whole scene you will be compelled to check the flow of that drop of water because it will worry you. But if you are very alert and totally non-judgemental, the sound will lead you to touch even deeper chords of your being. In other words, being non-judgemental means to see but not react.

3 Being in a relaxed state is a fundamental prerequisite for meditation. To reach that state of relaxation, you can sing, dance, jog, run, swim, walk, do yoga without trying to achieve anything from it because just the next step beyond relaxation is meditation. A feeling of ease and relaxation can be achieved by the mere acceptance of one's surroundings. You can realise this right now, wherever you might be. Just try it and feel the difference.

4 Don't hold on to beliefs. They will suffocate you because living with laws and so-called rights does not lead to happiness. Imagine being tied to a chain like a dog and told that you cannot go wrong now because you cannot move. Is happiness possible in this state? Having lived with all your beliefs for so long, you have become totally incapable of going beyond these boundaries that you have created for yourself. You fight just to live with them. How can you be free and happy by holding on to beliefs that consume your energy? By letting them go, you go beyond right and wrong. You are able respond to every situation in a different way, which is not based on

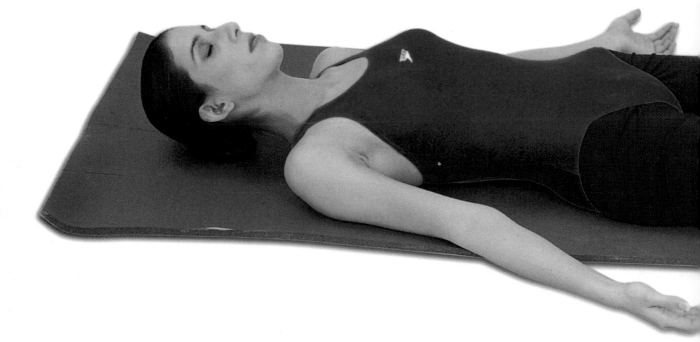

a predetermined law. Right is simply the ability of a man to perform an activity without guilt.

5 Only fearlessness can lead you to freedom. The basic mystery of man is that he wants to be free from all fears. Fear comes from a feeling of control, a feeling that there is nothing beyond oneself. But fear can only go in surrender, not in control. One should understand that nothing is really in our hands. And if this is so, then why be afraid. Who can harm you if you understand that you are already of someone. So drop your fears and accept your natural state of surrender. Freedom will be gifted to you, and only then can you be meditative.

6 Practise yoga till you reach a natural state of meditation. The whole purpose of yoga is to take you to a natural state of union of the body and the mind, and then take you to the third dimension of human consciousness. So to tap the higher channels of your being, you don't need more information or knowledge. You simply have to

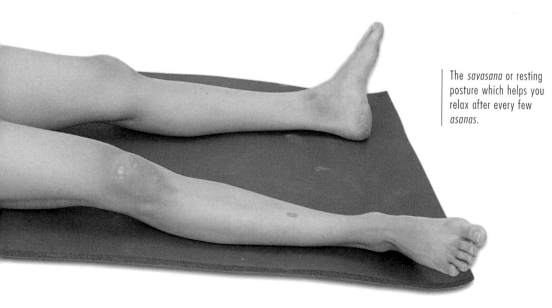

The *savasana* or resting posture which helps you relax after every few *asanas*.

be in that expanded state. Stop reading spiritual books on *charkas*, *nadis* and enlightenment. Or else, you might artificially create it in your mind. Avoid all trips of the mind.

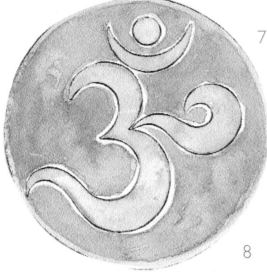

7 Only desirelessness can lead you to a meditative state. Desire means that you are not content as you are, right now. You feel your happiness lies in tomorrow. And that tomorrow will never come. Desire makes you live in a world called tomorrow. So you negate your present and base your existence on the illusion of tomorrow. Desirelessness is simply living in the present.

8 Don't try to concentrate. Yogis never talk about sitting down to meditate. Just start expanding in whatever you are doing. By concentration you only end up doing what you are not supposed to do at that point of time. For the rest of the time your life remains the same. Instead, bring your awareness and alertness to everything you do. Bring meditation into your life 24 hours a day, not just for twenty minutes or one hour.

The symbol Om (pronounced Auhm) is the last sound preceding total silence or meditation. Repeating this powerful mantra for fifteen minutes calms the mind and also energises the entire system.

9 Don't try to be perfect. Accept yourself as you are. Simply be a witness. Remain in a state of watchful awareness. Perfection is a man made concept, and godliness is simply a complete acceptance of yourself.

10 The singer has become the song. The painter has become the painting. This is what meditation is about. There is no object and no subject. They have become one.

Seven-day Schedule for General Fitness

Start with *surya namaskar* (sun salutation) every day. This warms and opens up your body, preparing you for the *asanas*. Now practise the *asanas* for the two body parts mentioned in the schedule. Working on specific body parts every day is more effective as two related muscle groups are targeted intensively. It also allows them to rest for the next two days. Practised this way, your progress will be more rapid. After the *asanas*, practise all the three *bandhas*. This is important as *bandhas* affect the hormonal system, which in turn affects the functioning of your whole body. Then practise one *kriya* to enrich your system with oxygen, and increase its basic metabolic rate (BMR). Practise one *pranayama* while sitting in a meditative posture. This will stabilise your breathing, relax the muscles and bring your body back to equilibrium. *Tratak kriya* can be practised as often as one wants, but not more than once a day.

Seven-day Schedule for General Fitness

Monday

Surya namaskar, asanas for sides and upper body, all three *bandhas* – *Jalandhar bandha, Udyan bandha, Mool bandha, Kapalbhati kriya, Sahaj pranayama*

Tuesday

Surya namaskar, asanas for abdomen and back, all three *bandhas* – *Jalandhar bandha, Udyan bandha, Mool bandha, Agnisar kriya, Sheetkari* or *Sheetli pranayama*

Wednesday

Surya namaskar, asanas for legs and hips, all three *bandhas* – *Jalandhar bandha, Udyan bandha, Mool bandha, Dhokan kriya, Anulom-Vilom pranayama*

Thursday

Surya namaskar, asanas for sides and upper body, all three *bandhas* – *Jalandhar bandha, Udyan bandha, Mool bandha, Kapalbhati kriya, Sahaj pranayama*

Friday

Surya namaskar, asanas for abdomen and back, all three *bandhas* – *Jalandhar bandha, Udyan bandha, Mool bandha, Agnisar kriya, Sheetkari* or *Sheetli pranayama*

Saturday

Surya namaskar, asanas for legs and hips, all three *bandhas* – *Jalandhar bandha, Udyan bandha, Mool bandha, Dhokan kriya, Anulom-Vilom pranayama*

Sunday

Surya namaskar, inverted postures and meditative postures

Curing Ailments
through Yoga

Yoga is not only excellent for general fitness but is also useful for alleviating and curing specific ailments. In this pictorial section special postures are given which help in some common problems from abdominal disorders and asthma to cervical spondylitis, diabetes and high blood pressure. Practise these *asanas* for your specific health problem, in addition to your daily schedule.

126

ANXIETY

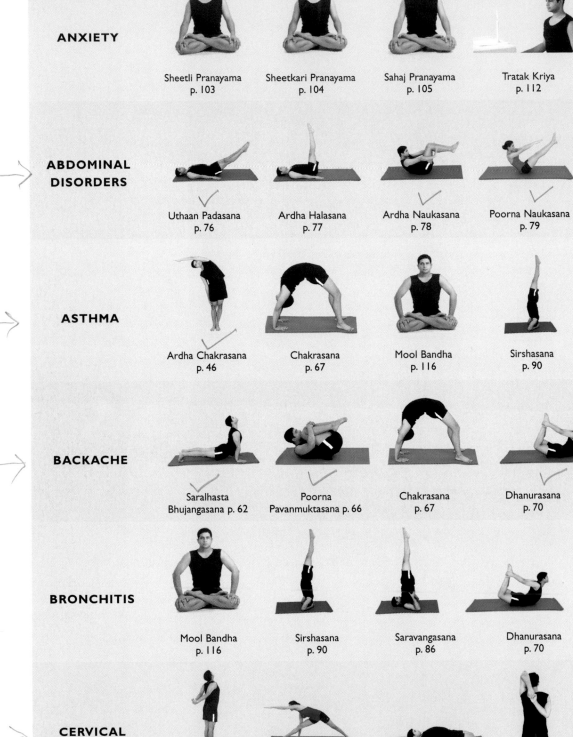

Sheetli Pranayama
p. 103

Sheetkari Pranayama
p. 104

Sahaj Pranayama
p. 105

Tratak Kriya
p. 112

Kapalbhati Kriya
p. 110

ABDOMINAL DISORDERS

Uthaan Padasana
p. 76

Ardha Halasana
p. 77

Ardha Naukasana
p. 78

Poorna Naukasana
p. 79

Kati Naukasana
p. 80

ASTHMA

Ardha Chakrasana
p. 46

Chakrasana
p. 67

Mool Bandha
p. 116

Sirshasana
p. 90

Saravangasana
p. 86

BACKACHE

Saralhasta
Bhujangasana p. 62

Poorna
Pavanmuktasana p. 66

Chakrasana
p. 67

Dhanurasana
p. 70

Dwikonasana
p. 74

BRONCHITIS

Mool Bandha
p. 116

Sirshasana
p. 90

Saravangasana
p. 86

Dhanurasana
p. 70

Saralhasta
Bhujangasana p. 62

CERVICAL SPONDYLITIS

Dwikonasana
p. 74

Uthitatrikonasana
p. 52

Supta Vajrasana
p. 31

Gomukhasana
p. 55

Virpritkarnimudra
p. 84

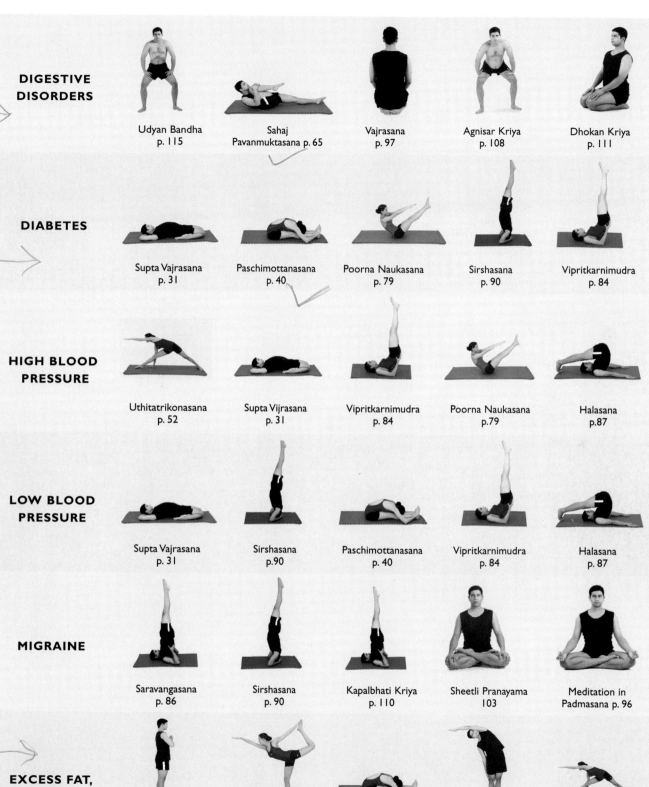

DIGESTIVE DISORDERS

Udyan Bandha
p. 115

Sahaj
Pavanmuktasana p. 65

Vajrasana
p. 97

Agnisar Kriya
p. 108

Dhokan Kriya
p. 111

DIABETES

Supta Vajrasana
p. 31

Paschimottanasana
p. 40

Poorna Naukasana
p. 79

Sirshasana
p. 90

Vipritkarnimudra
p. 84

HIGH BLOOD PRESSURE

Uthitatrikonasana
p. 52

Supta Vijrasana
p. 31

Vipritkarnimudra
p. 84

Poorna Naukasana
p.79

Halasana
p.87

LOW BLOOD PRESSURE

Supta Vajrasana
p. 31

Sirshasana
p.90

Paschimottanasana
p. 40

Vipritkarnimudra
p. 84

Halasana
p. 87

MIGRAINE

Saravangasana
p. 86

Sirshasana
p. 90

Kapalbhati Kriya
p. 110

Sheetli Pranayama
103

Meditation in
Padmasana p. 96

EXCESS FAT, OBESITY

Surya Namaskar
p. 20

Vatayanasana
p. 38

Paschimottanasana
p. 40

Ardha Chakrasana
p. 46

Uthitatrikonasana
p. 52

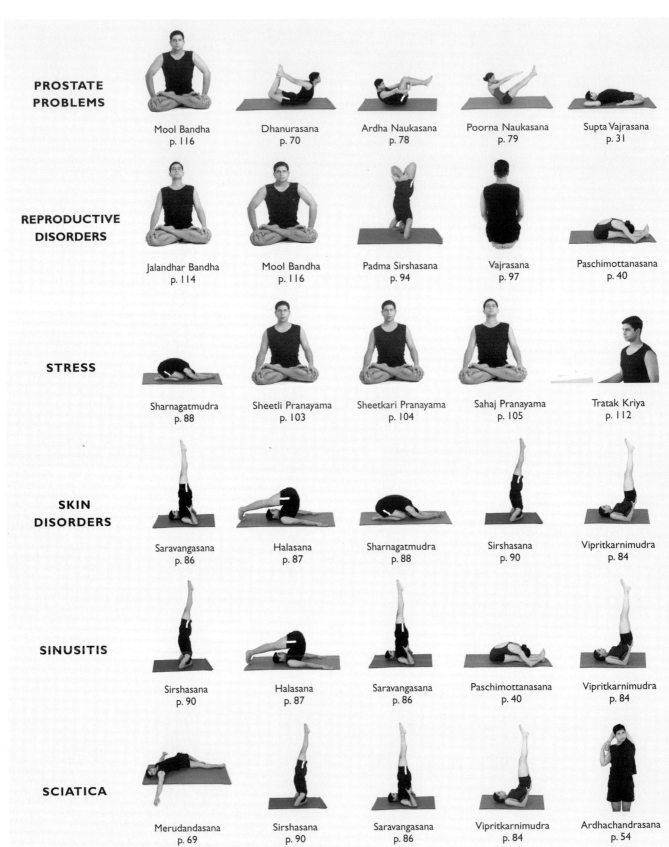

PROSTATE PROBLEMS

Mool Bandha
p. 116

Dhanurasana
p. 70

Ardha Naukasana
p. 78

Poorna Naukasana
p. 79

Supta Vajrasana
p. 31

REPRODUCTIVE DISORDERS

Jalandhar Bandha
p. 114

Mool Bandha
p. 116

Padma Sirshasana
p. 94

Vajrasana
p. 97

Paschimottanasana
p. 40

STRESS

Sharnagatmudra
p. 88

Sheetli Pranayama
p. 103

Sheetkari Pranayama
p. 104

Sahaj Pranayama
p. 105

Tratak Kriya
p. 112

SKIN DISORDERS

Saravangasana
p. 86

Halasana
p. 87

Sharnagatmudra
p. 88

Sirshasana
p. 90

Vipritkarnimudra
p. 84

SINUSITIS

Sirshasana
p. 90

Halasana
p. 87

Saravangasana
p. 86

Paschimottanasana
p. 40

Vipritkarnimudra
p. 84

SCIATICA

Merudandasana
p. 69

Sirshasana
p. 90

Saravangasana
p. 86

Vipritkarnimudra
p. 84

Ardhachandrasana
p. 54